Intermittent Fasting and Keto

The Ultimate Guide to IF for Women Who Want to Lose Weight, Burn Fat, and Increase Mental Clarity + A Guide to the Ketogenic Diet for Beginners

© Copyright 2019

All Rights Reserved. No part of this book may be reproduced in any form without permission in writing from the author. Reviewers may quote brief passages in reviews.

Disclaimer: No part of this publication may be reproduced or transmitted in any form or by any means, mechanical or electronic, including photocopying or recording, or by any information storage and retrieval system, or transmitted by email without permission in writing from the publisher.

While all attempts have been made to verify the information provided in this publication, neither the author nor the publisher assumes any responsibility for errors, omissions or contrary interpretations of the subject matter herein.

This book is for entertainment purposes only. The views expressed are those of the author alone, and should not be taken as expert instruction or commands. The reader is responsible for his or her own actions.

Adherence to all applicable laws and regulations, including international, federal, state and local laws governing professional licensing, business practices, advertising and all other aspects of doing business in the US, Canada, UK or any other jurisdiction is the sole responsibility of the purchaser or reader.

Neither the author nor the publisher assumes any responsibility or liability whatsoever on the behalf of the purchaser or reader of these materials. Any perceived slight of any individual or organization is purely unintentional.

Contents

PART 1: INTERMITTENT FASTING FOR WOMEN 0

INTRODUCTION 1

CHAPTER 1: WHAT IS INTERMITTENT FASTING? 5

CHAPTER 2: SCIENTIFIC BENEFITS OF INTERMITTENT FASTING .11

INTERMITTENT FASTING: WOMEN VERSUS MEN 15

CHAPTER 3: HOW FASTING IMPACTS WEIGHT LOSS 18

KETOSIS 22

CHAPTER 4: DIFFERENT INTERMITTENT FASTING TECHNIQUES .25

THE 16/8 METHOD 26

THE 5/2 DIET METHOD 27

THE EAT STOP EAT METHOD 27

THE ALTERNATING DAY METHOD 28

THE WARRIOR METHOD 28

THE SPONTANEITY METHOD 29

CUSTOMIZATION TECHNIQUES 29

    ☐ *Customization Strategy #1* *30*

    ☐ *Customization Strategy #2* *30*

    ☐ *Customization Strategy #3* *30*

    ☐ *Customization strategy #4* *31*

- *Customization strategy #5* *31*

CHAPTER 5: FASTING AND EXERCISE MYTHS EXPLAINED 33
- INTERMITTENT FASTING WILL SLOW YOUR METABOLISM 34
- BY JUST FASTING YOU WILL LOSE WEIGHT 34
- YOU CAN EAT ANYTHING YOU WANT IN BETWEEN FASTS 34
- INTERMITTENT FASTING IS EFFECTIVE AND EVERYONE SEES RESULTS 34
- FASTING IS STARVING YOURSELF AND UNHEALTHY 35
- FASTING LEADS TO MUSCLE LOSS 35
- EXERCISING LEADS TO WEIGHT LOSS 35
- THE BEST TIME TO EXERCISE IS IN THE MORNING 36
- EXERCISE BENEFITS ONLY THE PHYSICAL 36
- FASTED WORKOUTS 36
  - *Yoga* *38*
  - *Tai Chi* *38*
  - *Jogging* *39*
  - *Cardio* *39*
  - *Pilates* *40*
  - *Hiking* *40*

CHAPTER 6: BEST FOODS FOR FASTING 41
- LEAFY GREENS 43
- GARLIC 44
- POTATOES 44
- TOMATOES 44
- BROCCOLI 44
- CAULIFLOWER 44
- SUNFLOWER SEEDS 45
- ALMONDS 45
- BLUEBERRIES 45
- RASPBERRIES 45

- CHOCOLATE 45
- BEANS 46
- RICE 46
- TOFU 46
- SALMON 46
- SHELLFISH 46
- MEAL PREPPING 47
  - *Breakfast* *49*
  - *Lunch* *51*
  - *Dinner* *52*
  - ☐ *Whole* *53*
  - *Snacks* *54*
- NOTABLE DIETS 54
  - *Mediterranean Diet* *55*
  - *Paleo Diet* *55*
  - *Ketogenic Diets* *56*
  - *Vegetarian Diets* *57*
  - *Vegan Diet* *58*
  - *The Whole30 Diet* *58*
  - *Raw Food Diet* *58*

CHAPTER 7: GETTING STARTED 60

CHAPTER 8: ONE WEEK STEP-BY-STEP GUIDE 64

- THE 16/8 METHOD 65
  - *Guideline:* *65*
  - *Sunday* *65*
  - *Key Points:* *66*
  - *Monday (Day 1)* *66*
  - *Tuesday (Day 2)* *67*
  - *Wednesday (Day 3)* *68*

    Thursday (Day 4) *68*

    Friday (Day 5) *69*

    Saturday (Day 6) *70*

    Sunday (Day 7) *70*

THE 5/2 METHOD 71

    Sunday *71*

    Monday (Day 1) *72*

    Tuesday (Day 2) *73*

    Wednesday (Day 3) *73*

    Thursday (Day 4) *74*

    Friday (Day 5) *74*

    Saturday (Day 6) *74*

    Sunday (Day 7) *75*

THE EAT STOP EAT METHOD 75

    Sunday *75*

    Monday (Day 1) *76*

    Tuesday (Day 2) *77*

    Wednesday (Day 3) *78*

    Thursday (Day 4) *78*

    Friday (Day 5) *78*

    Saturday (Day 6) *79*

    Sunday (Day 7) *79*

    Added Notes on the Eat Stop Eat Method *79*

ALTERNATE DAY METHOD 79

    Sunday *80*

    Monday (Day 1) *80*

    Tuesday (Day 2) *80*

    Wednesday (Day 3) *81*

    Thursday (Day 4) *81*

  Friday (Day 5) *82*

  Saturday (Day 6) *82*

  Sunday (Day 7) *82*

 WARRIOR METHOD 83

  Sunday *83*

  Monday (Day 1) *83*

  Tuesday (Day 2) *84*

  Wednesday (Day 3) *85*

  Thursday (Day 4) *85*

  Friday (Day 5) *86*

  Saturday (Day 6) *86*

  Sunday (Day 7) *86*

 SPONTANEITY METHOD 87

CHAPTER 9: DOS AND DON'TS OF INTERMITTENT FASTING **89**

CONCLUSION **94**

PART 2: KETO DIET **96**

INTRODUCTION **97**

CHAPTER 1: THE BEGINNING **98**

 TYPES OF KETO DIETS 100

  Standard Ketogenic Diet *100*

  High-Protein Ketogenic Diet *101*

  Cyclical Ketogenic Diet *101*

  Targeted Ketogenic Diet *101*

 THE TRUTH ABOUT CARBS 102

 WHAT MAKES US FAT 103

 MYTHBUSTING WITH THE KETO DIET 103

 WHY SHOULD YOU DO THE KETO DIET 106

 COMMON MISTAKES KETO BEGINNERS MAKE 109

 VISITING A DIETICIAN (OR A NUTRITIONIST) 113

CHAPTER 2: KETONES 116
    GET YOURSELF INTO KETOSIS 116
    HOW TO KNOW WHEN YOU'RE IN KETOSIS 118
    TESTS 120
    KETONE SUPPLEMENTS 121

CHAPTER 3: BENEFITS OF KETOSIS 123
    THE BAD EFFECT OF TOO MUCH SUGAR 126
    THE TRUTH ABOUT THE "DANGERS" OF LOW-CARB DIETS 128

CHAPTER 4: MACROS 131
    CARBS 132
    PROTEIN 133
    FATS 133
    MEASURING YOUR CALORIES AND MACROS 134
        Your Basal Metabolic Rate 135
        Your Total Daily Energy Expenditure 136
        Your Body Fat Percentage 137
        Men 138
        Women 139
    ADJUSTING YOUR CALORIE INTAKE 140
        Carb Intake 141
        Protein 142
        Fats 142

CHAPTER 5: NUTRITION 144
    MEATS 144
    FATS AND OILS 145
    VEGETABLES 146
    DAIRY 148
    NUTS AND SEEDS 150
    SEAFOOD 151

 BERRIES 152

 EGGS 153

 SAUCES 153

 DRINKS 154

 SEVEN-DAY MEAL PLAN 155

  Day 1 ....*155*

  Day 2 ....*155*

  Day 3 ....*156*

  Day 4 ....*156*

  Day 5 ....*156*

  Day 6 ....*157*

  Day 7 ....*157*

  Bulletproof Coffee *157*

  Foods That Are Off Limits *158*

  Easy Substitutions for Foods *160*

 MEAL PREP FOR BEGINNERS 163

 TO-DO LIST 164

CHAPTER 6: THE KETO FLU 166

 SUGAR CRAVINGS 168

CHAPTER 7: EXERCISING 171

CHAPTER 8: SOCIALIZING 174

 ALCOHOL 177

 ACTIVITIES TO DO WITH FRIENDS (THAT DON'T INVOLVE EATING OR DRINKING) 181

 LIVING WITH THOSE WHO AREN'T INTO KETO 185

 CHEATING ON KETO 186

 GETTING BACK ON TRACK 190

CHAPTER 9: YOU AND KETO 191

 BE PERSISTENT 193

STAY MOTIVATED	193
MAKE SMALL CHANGES	194
DON'T USE FOOD AS REWARDS	195
CONTROL EMOTIONAL EATING	195
PRACTICE MINDFUL EATING	196
CONCLUSION	**197**

Part 1: Intermittent Fasting for Women

An Essential Guide to Weight Loss, Fat-Burning, and Healing Your Body Without Sacrificing All Your Favorite Foods

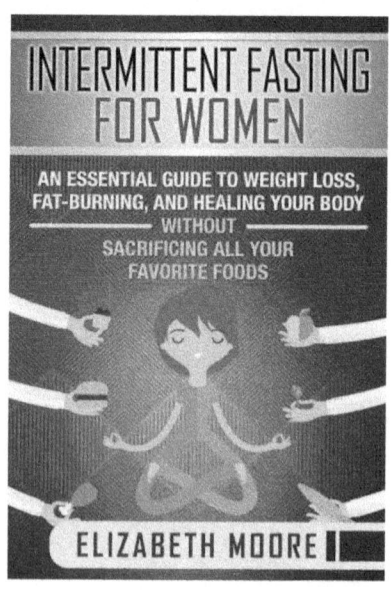

Introduction

This book is dedicated to the individual who wishes to improve her life through the transformative practice of Intermittent Fasting and weight loss. We will explore and discover what it takes to truly transform our day-to-day life into a positive and beneficial lifestyle, not only by simply cutting out some meals here and there but also by taking time to examine our habits, analyze our life choices up to this point, and be truthful with ourselves about our bodies and minds. This is not a casual diet fad manifesto but an immersive guideline to successful and safe weight loss. What it takes to cut weight and keep it off does not have to involve quitting your favorite foods and guilty pleasures, although it will require discipline, confidence, and a true desire to transform your life for the better. This well-rounded book is not a miracle cure for problems but a book that presents methods to transform your body and mindset. Your outlook on life is just as important as physical health, and here, we will explore the relationship between the two.

Transformation is the most important word in this book. We will aim to keep transformation as the key goal – not only the transformation of our diet or health but a transformation of our entire lives. If this seems too far out of reach, do not be discouraged – it is easier than you think. Transformation does not require us to change who we truly are. We can keep all the things we love, but it will require a rewiring of how we view ourselves and the world around us. What could normally trigger a negative or detrimental attitude will be altered and viewed from a different perspective, a perspective that comes from a place of self-love and confidence. By applying the knowledge and practices we are about to learn into our lives, we can develop a lifestyle that will become second nature and only help us stay healthful physically and mentally.

In the chapters to come, we will discuss the ins and outs of Intermittent Fasting with an emphasis on women's weight loss in today's busy and complicated world. Women have had to battle more difficulties than men for all of written history, and today is no different. Naturally, the extra stress on women to look and behave a certain way makes it very difficult to maintain balance during the mundane day-to-day tasks, thus making healthful lifestyles a choice that is overlooked or flat out cannot be obtained. All the fad diets and exercise cannot extinguish centuries of struggle, no, but taking care of our bodies on an individual level while navigating the tough social terrain is a step in the right direction to health and happiness. No technology or wonder drug will ever be the miracle cure it's claiming to be, but creating a wonderful life and feeling amazing doesn't have to be difficult. In fact, the path to balanced health comes with a few simple changes in the way we treat food and ourselves. We need to reevaluate the social norms and their detrimental effect on our lifestyles. We need to filter out the noise of our fast-paced lifestyles and redesign our eating habits to benefit each of us as an individual. There is no end all be all solution to great health; our bodies and our world are constantly changing, and we need to change with it.

With the advent of modified foods and advanced science, our current society seems to work efficiently. Our technological progress has provided luxuries beyond the fantasies of the population that thrived only a couple of hundred years ago, but there are still problems pertaining to the influence on our health with these advancements. Travel technology, accompanied by a globe completely interconnected by the Internet, has allowed cultures to cross-pollinate. Rich foods from all around the world are accessible for the first time, but so is overconsumption. The luxuries of fast food and processed snacks have paved the way for our society of diversity and information to turn to quick satisfaction rather than mindful consumption, this inevitably turning into a weight gain problem in our society.

As services and goods become easier to acquire, less emphasis and attention is given to our bodies and minds. We replace healthful lifestyles with the laziest ones. Food becomes simply something we "drive-thru" a tiny window for, time set aside for exercise takes a back seat to social media, and instead of mindfulness, we find ourselves zombie-like and nullified. Obesity and excessive weight gain are abundant, and confidence in ourselves seems to be at an all-time low. As the current structure slips away into a health crisis, there are things that individuals can do to counteract the negative effects, no matter how lazy you are.

This is where Intermittent Fasting (IF) comes into play. Although a practice used regularly by ancient cultures and indigenous ones today, fasting has become much more popular in contemporary culture in recent years. Fasting is the intentional cutting off of caloric intake to benefit the body and mind. Intermittent Fasting is cutting off caloric intake for a predetermined set part of the day – that is, only eating for a respected window of hours. Not eating throughout the day may sound like no fun at first, and the mere thought of the starving feeling is discomforting, and it may be, at first, but through a dedicated practice of Intermittent Fasting, we give rise to a new feeling, one of empowerment and control. Many were raised to believe that the ideal diet is having three square meals a day and plenty of snacks in between, but the science and visible results prevail as our society embraces the practice and fasting finds its way into our daily lives.

Intermittent Fasting is a simple and very effective way not only to lose weight safely and naturally but also keeps the mind sharp by creating a distinct awareness of the food we take for granted every day. By cutting caloric intake for certain times of the day, we find a more structured eating plan, one that the body benefits from as you cut unnecessary weight while also benefitting the brain by changing the way we look at meals. These benefits balance the mind-body experience, building new relationships with food, health, and ourselves. The balance of body and mind is the best preventative measure to ensure that we feel amazing every day, awake refreshed, and live our lives to the fullest.

If you are reading this, you've no doubt tried many other techniques to lose weight and feel great. If you have been frightened away from fasting because it's been presented as extreme or unhealthy, do not worry. In this book, we will focus on the key elements of Intermittent Fasting and how it can help women lose weight while not changing their lives completely. In the chapters to come, we will focus heavily on Intermittent Fasting as a path to transformation of the body and mind. The reason we choose to view this as a transformative practice is simple: we want to treat ourselves not as only scientific explanations and results but as powerful beings that are capable of taking control of their lives and transforming them. When seeing our bodies through this lens, we can visualize the results of our practice, motivating ourselves to achieve these goals. Mindfulness and awareness are key components to weight loss and an amazing life in general.

In this book, we aim to present methods of fasting that can be easily customized to fit your schedule. We will explore the science and safety of Intermittent Fasting, suitable foods, and dietary guidelines, and how safely to exercise while fasting. This is a transformational path not only of the body but of the mind and perception of health.

You may not have discovered the right material that presents the practice in an appealing way, but rest assured that this book is for you. Let's begin this journey with an open mind and open heart as we introduce Intermittent Fasting to our lives.

Chapter 1: What is Intermittent Fasting?

Let's get right to the point. Fasting is a relatively simple practice that yields incredible and complicated results. The effects that fasting has on the body and mind seem unfathomable: weight loss, blood sugar regulation, blood pressure regulation, and growth hormone regulation – only to name a few important ones. In recent years, science has come full force to support these claims, not to mention the thousands of videos online of people's results now that fasting has hit the mainstream. There are different types of fasting as well as many ways to fast.

Within the abundant array of different methods and individual changes any one person may implement, there is a wealth of potential ways to impact the health of the body and mind in positive ways. Fasting, in a general and broad definition, is the practice of willingly abstaining from something, usually food and drink. Whether it is simply not eating chocolate for a week or two or even cutting out all solid foods for a month, no matter how large or small the impact the abstinence has on you, that is fasting from your chosen food. Another more intensive fast would be dry fasting. Dry fasting is the complete abstinence from every source of solid or liquid food for any predetermined period, and, of course, willingly. Although not completely out of the question for beginners, these styles of fasting are used more sparingly than the style we aim to focus on, and that practice is called Intermittent Fasting or IF for short.

IF is very similar to the practices described above, but instead of completely fasting for days at a time, you would choose a certain time of the day, say an eight-hour period. This time window would be the only time you ingest foods as much as you'd like depending on your personal goals. There may also be other rules you set yourself, but there's more on customizing your practice later in the book. The idea of intentionally choosing not to eat may be contradictory to many of the views on food that our culture holds dear. Abundance and indulgence run rampant in our world, and the more you have, the better, right? Not so much. As we now see the results of the destructive habits we have formed, we must look to other answers, better practices, and mindful analyzation of what and when we eat. Changing our eating habit is no small feat; it takes a strong will and a desire to attain a more meaningful and healthy life, one that is not overburdened with sugary snacks and stress caused by overeating. As we can see, IF is not so much a new fad diet but a distinct and progressive lifestyle choice. And although these practices have only recently hit the mainstream in our world today, there is a long and fruitful lineage of practices from cultures all around the world that practiced fasting, and we look to these cultures and our distant ancestors for inspiration and guidance on this journey.

Before today's fast-paced society took hold of our diets, fasting played a very important role in essentially every culture and society around the world. Whether it was for spiritual purposes, health reasons, or some intense ritual, fasting was a lynchpin in many lifestyles throughout human history. Even before humans had science to explore the details of how our bodies work on a microscopic level, we knew that fasting was a source of good health and wellbeing. Primitive cultures would often require fasting before battles and even as an initiatory milestone during puberty. The prehistorical humans surely weren't as concerned about their weight and appearances as we are now, but the hunter-gatherer lifestyle would seemingly fit nicely within the scope of IF. Wandering place to place in search of nutrients, there may have been plenty of time in between meals, but is this fasting? Sure, the ancient tribes probably went long periods without food but probably not willingly. It's impossible to truly find out what the ancient cultures were thinking and practicing, but here, we see potential caloric restriction that influenced early man in incredible ways, perhaps even influencing the onset of agriculture and settling.

As humans progressed and began settling, we see a more prominent and definitive practice of fasting. We see all the big hitters in the religious world advocating for it; Jesus Christ, Muhammed, and Buddha all viewed fasting as a purification process. Commonly based on religious grounds, fasting became a practice of sacrifice, giving up something to show a respected god or entity that you were devoted and deserved good graces from powerful beings. The idea of giving up something so precious, which was required to survive, would surely appease the gods. Certainly, as these practices caught on, the humans, religious or not, felt the results of their fasts. Fasting stays a prominent aspect of medicine as the timeline progresses onward into some ancient cultures that we have better historical documentation of.

The ancient Greek philosophers valued fasting among their other important contributions to our current world. Hippocrates, the father of modern medicine, focused heavily on fasting for a balanced and healthful life. He spoke and promoted the practice while also prescribing it to his patients. The Greek philosophy drew heavily from nature; the observation that humans lose their appetite when they are sick showed the Greek philosophers and doctors that the body naturally restricts caloric intake when ill, and thus there must be some value to the healing potential of willingly abstaining from caloric intake. Another father of contemporary medicine who advocated for fasting was Paracelsus, the inventor of toxicology. He wrote, "Fasting is the greatest remedy, the physician within." The reference to "the physician within" alludes to the body having a natural ability to intuitively heal itself, let alone have assistance by the human mind through the willingness to abstain and attention to the nuances of the mind-body connection. These ancient ideas helped build the foundation of our current state of medicine, but perhaps we need to return to the ideas held dear to our ancestors.

While considering that our ancient ancestors and some of the most prominent minds of our time utilized IF as a means of attaining optimal health, we look forward to today's world. Although the Western world relies heavily on processed foods and a constant intake of foods throughout the day, many contemporary societies live quite the opposite and thrive just as well or even better. One example that stands out is the Hunzakuts of Northern Pakistan. Thriving in the Hunza valley, these people are well known to live well past one hundred years of age, even documenting one woman who was 130 years old! Along with this incredible longevity, the Hunza are living without hardly any degenerative disease. With their diets being high in mineral content and low in sodium, their longevity can be attributed to this, but there is another key factor that suits our purposes. The Hunza people have a very limited food intake. Even without the complicated science and meal plans, they have withheld a standard of longevity quite naturally. Their recent history before being touched by civilization had very interesting patterns that they adhered to not out of choice but simply because that was how they lived their lives. The Hunza people's annual harvest each year would be exhausted, and they would live with minimal caloric intake for weeks at a time each spring. Once the last year's food supply was depleted, they would have minimal sustenance until the new harvest began. With more modern science showing that limited caloric intake has amazing effects on the body and brain, as we will explore, the longevity of the Hunza is linked to their IF lifestyle, along with their distinct diet.

So, around the world, we see fasting being used for survival and necessity, but what about fasting for other purposes? IF finds itself permeating so many aspects of our culture that it cannot be ignored as a key element in human life and survival.

Today, we see fasting prominent in the most widely practiced religions. These holidays and traditions permeate all of the cultures in our interconnected world. Ramadan is a holy month in Islamic religions, during the ninth month of their calendar adherents fast from dawn to dusk – this is IF at its core. Christianity has its holy fast called Lent. This six-week period begins on Ash Wednesday and ends on Easter Sunday, where during this time, there are many celebrations and practices, but fasting remains a very important aspect. For Jewish cultures, Yom Kippur stands out as an important fast day, comprised of a 25-hour fast and intensive prayer. These examples being the most popular, let's not forget that all religions and cultures use fasting. The non-religious and more fact-based mind benefit from fasting's rigorous power to change and alter health. Mahatma Gandhi famously undertook seventeen fasts while fighting for India's independence, showing that fasting isn't simply for health or religious benefit, but can be used to usher in revolution and political change. However, what about all of us who aren't religious adherents or world-changing revolutionaries?

The history of fasting lays a solid foundation that cannot be ignored in modern times. New science technology is confirming the history and reassuring contemporary populations that IF is a safe, effective, and simple path to overall health. Not only is fasting resting comfortably on the shoulders of science and history, but it also has perks in the consumerist world we live in. Since fasting requires no prescriptions, no fitness contraptions, and no expensive supplements, the practice fits nicely within our money-hungry, materialist society. Simply abstaining from something you love to eat for a day or two changes your outlook on your potential to take control of your life and literally will save you money as you will be consuming less than usual. As practical as it sounds, many feel that it is too good to be true, that simply not eating could not possibly affect the body and brain as much as people claim. And sure, at first glance, it seems like a gimmick that celebrity doctors want to scam you with, but given the test of time and solid science, fasting will remain a pivotal practice in the rearranging of our lives in the Western world, an action that desperately needs to be put into play.

Now that we've gotten acquainted with the history and basics of fasting and its role in our society let's focus on some in-depth science on IF to truly grasp what will happen when we begin this amazing journey of transformation.

Chapter 2: Scientific Benefits of Intermittent Fasting

Relying on the knowledge of ancient cultures grants a certain amount of philosophical insight but is limited in the scientific background our twenty-first-century minds require to be rest assured. Fortunately, many studies on IF are popping up all over the Internet, with sound scientific evidence that fasting is as safe and effective, if not more so than any other diet that hits the mainstream. For decades, we have thought that what we eat is the most important aspect of whether or not our diets are considered healthy. However, many other factors are in play. Not only what we eat, but how it's prepared, where it's sourced, and when we eat. These combined with physical and mental exercise create our state of health, and IF affects all of these aspects.

By taking on an IF routine, we funnel our view of food and meals through a new lens, thus transforming our mindset about food and the food we ingest and when. This transformation has been shown to increase self-worth, while simultaneously reduce stress, which on a psychological level is incredibly beneficial for someone looking to lose weight. Let's keep this positive outlook and confidence in mind as we approach IF from a strictly scientific perspective.

In a very broad sense, IF's physical results are attributed to calorie restriction. It makes sense, right? Eat less, get thin. But it goes deeper than this simple equation. Lab studies have shown that calorie restriction has been attributed to the reduction of illnesses related to death and lengthened lifespans. Studies have shown that in mice obesity, the risk of metabolic diseases are lowered due to caloric restriction – these reactions having been also proven to translate to humans. Not only can the restrictions help prevent obesity, but they were also shown to reset circadian rhythms and balance the rhythm of hormonal secretions. These rhythms, of which there are many, keep our body in check, ensuring that our body is running smoothly and efficiently. This biological rhythm is very apparent when a fast begins. The rhythm of your digestive system becomes very clear while fasting. Since digestion is essentially 'turned off' once we go to bed, it is subsequently turned back on the moment we intake calories the next morning. So, if we restrict calorie intake, our digestive system will rest until we eat again; while it rests, it repairs itself. By giving our systems plenty of time to repair in between meals, we achieve a simple yet effective and concise practice that assists our body with its natural healing methods. With IF and assigning a strict consumption window, we can actively engage with our natural digestive rhythm, keeping it in sync with the rest of our body as we see fit. The digestive system seems to be an obvious player in weight loss, but what about the control center and epic organ, the human brain?

The human brain is mysterious and complicated; science has certainly only scratched the surface of what must be an infinite amount of investigation into the brain. As the 'control center' of our entire body, it plays a major role in weight loss. The brain not only influences the physical aspects of the body, hormone regulation, and autonomous actions like breathing and blood pumping, but also more in-depth metaphysical ideas, like thought and emotion, are considered to be housed in the brain to some extent. As mysterious as it is, we will stand with these claims. And so, our ideas will play a huge role in our IF journey, and a positive outlook and practicing confidence-building affirmations will go hand in hand with the fasting experience. So consider the brain an avenue for thought and emotion. You are in control and IF will help you come to this realization.

We've spent our whole lives thinking and believing that the societal structure of diets and foods are the most efficient. We need to break from these patterns and do what is best for us individually. Again, no one way of living will work for everyone. On the scientific level, we send signals to our brain that allow it to regulate and restore where need be. So, naturally, if you were to eat less or not eat when you normally do, the brain will assume that the food is scarce and will take the necessary actions. Although the brain may reduce the metabolic rate and attempt to conserve fat reserves, it is still burning reserved fat instead of recently ingested sugars, combined with suitable exercise (found later in the book). This is a very effective and safe weight loss strategy. However, let's not forget that the brain will also start releasing growth hormones to regulate and account for new changes in diet and routine. These are hormones that have been shown to increase longevity and reduce the effects of aging. The brain isn't the only organ that responds positively to IF though.

Many wonder about the idea of the heart being the center of love and emotion. The symbolic idea of the heart is timeless, but what role can it play in our IF journey? The heart regulates blood flow, then the blood distributes nutrients and antibodies to all parts of the body. Considering the major causes of heart disease – cholesterol, blood pressure, weight, and diabetes – we find studies that show how IF assists in balancing all these bodily functions. The influence that this kind of fasting can have on these functions is important. As mentioned before, IF can help reset and assist the body to heal naturally. So, in turn, fasting helps regulate and balance these functions, then fasting directly influences the heart and its major enemies. We will discuss later in the book the potential risks of fasting, but here, we would like to state that some cases have found that extensive fasting can be attributed to electrolyte imbalances, which could affect the heart in negative ways.

The third major organ we want to focus on is the liver. The liver acts as a filtration system for the body while also producing bile to be sent to the intestines. As the filtration system, the liver will play a key role in the positive effects of IF. The caloric restriction itself acts as a symbolic representation of purification while quite literally not consuming any foods for a prolonged period will assist the liver in repairing itself. One particular study also shows us that when calories are restricted, the liver secretes a protein that adjusts the liver's metabolism. The regulation of the metabolism is key in producing weight loss results, and as we've seen, fasting interacts with the metabolism on many levels.

The science that has dedicated itself to fasting has shown what many believed for centuries before computers – that fasting is an all-around beneficial practice for overall wellbeing. Along with the three major organs discussed above, some key points should be emphasized:

- It gives the body more energy by assisting in the creation of mitochondria, which are power sources within every cell of your body. This gives you the energy that is used throughout the body. Having more energy will only assist in keeping up regular exercise and daily duties.
- It boosts growth hormone secretions in the brain. Although available in supplements, wouldn't human growth hormones (HGH) be more effective naturally occurring in the brain? By fasting, we increase the levels secreted by the brain, thus taking advantage of the hormone's natural ability to slow the effects of aging, improve cognitive performance, and protect the brain's health overall.
- It and its caloric restrictions allow the body to burn up stored fat rather than sugars. Fat is a cleaner source of energy than carbs or sugars and reduces inflammation by lowering

free radical production, and free radicals are thought to oxidize cells which could lead to autoimmune diseases and the like.
- It reduces inflammation which is attributed to many common diseases, such as dementia and obesity. Inflammation damages cells and IF helps to clean away the damaged cells. Ketones are produced through the burning of fat instead of sugar, and they regulate inflammation. IF also helps the body not become resistant to insulin. Insulin can potentially build up in the blood and create inflammation.

With the incredible effects that IF presents, it is no wonder that it was common amongst our ancestors and now common in the mainstream during the twenty-first century. We know through this science that IF can help us on so many levels, but what about our main goal with this book – weight loss? If we are to focus on shedding some pounds, we need to look deeper into the specific effects that this kind of fasting has on our excess fat and body image as a whole.

Intermittent Fasting: Women Versus Men

There is much debate about the different effects that IF has on women versus the effects that men experience. Although quite similar in many ways, there are distinct differences in the chemistry that makes up the different genders. Even when it comes to fasting, women should approach the practice a little differently than men.

Some studies show that low-energy diets can negatively affect fertility in women. The evolutionary nature of the female body to monitor and tune in to any threats to fertility makes the decreased supply of food and nutrients a huge red flag to the intuition of the woman's body. The sensitivity of women's hormonal balance is directly related to caloric intake and energy supply. In the past, body fat percentage was thought to be the key factor when it came to drastic hormonal changes, but now it is understood that energy, in general, plays a huge role as well. As for IF, the hormonal changes are the body's reactions to environmental conditions being altered, as we've discussed, so this combined with women can result in heightened sensitivity to changes.

There have been some documented cases of women missing menstrual cycles, experiencing drastic metabolic disruption, and uncontrollable binge eating during fasting routines. While these experiences are incredibly rare, it's important to take into account that the human body is mysterious, and many people have completely different experiences under very similar circumstances. So when considering an IF routine, we need to take great caution and listen to our bodies closely if we choose to go through with the practice.

What causes such rare side effects stem from the environmental influence that stimulates the hormonal glands in the brain. These glands – hypothalamus, pituitary, and gonadal – work together to regulate hormones that act on the reproductive organs. This leads us to conclude that when the precise and specific cycle needed to regulate the hormones is disrupted, it could have adverse effects. Why this seems to occur more often to women rather than men is unknown. There is speculation about a particular molecule called kisspeptin that may contribute to this phenomenon. Although kisspeptin exists in both male and female bodies, there is much more of it in women. This molecule may be the culprit, but it is until undetermined.

With what we know about the effects on fertility, we need to take into consideration the role that metabolism plays in all this. Metabolism and fertility work together to benefit each other in many ways. So if the hormones are being disrupted, physical reactions in the body can be concerning. Another topic of debate is the fact that women typically consume less protein than men. So, while fasting, there's an intake of less protein, and less protein is going to mean less amino acids, which are needed to stimulate estrogen receptors.

Again, we see the hormonal faculties being potentially disrupted by taking on an IF routine. While we need to keep this in mind, these rare occurrences shouldn't scare you away from fasting completely. However, if you experience any of the following conditions while fasting, you should end the fast as soon as possible. Break your fast if you experience the following:

- Irregular menstrual cycle
- Hair loss
- Wild mood swings
- Noticeable digestive irregularities
- Feeling abnormal and consistent cold
- Extreme intolerance to stress

As we take these potential side effects on IF into consideration, we also need to consider the fact that it is not for everyone. While the practice is very effective for some people, not everyone is going to enjoy fasting, let alone find benefits in the practice if they simply aren't built for it. If you would describe yourself as unhealthy or new to exercise, then fasting should be preceded by dietary changes and casual exercise. This will prepare your body for the fast and act to reduce shock on your body. Any eating disorders should be dealt with extreme care when approaching fasting as well. And, of course, women who are pregnant should not fast at all.

While women need a little more nuance and attention to detail when considering IF compared to men, we need not let this discourage us from our intended goals in this book. If anything, the complexity of the female body should be an attribute we find intriguing and beautiful, rather than assuming women's complexity is a hindrance. The main rule is to listen to your body, be aware of your changes, and build a relationship with your body. If you find that IF is not going to work for you, you can still gain much from this book. Taking the ideas and methods that we will explore in subsequent chapters can be modified to suit any path with a little alteration and thought.

Chapter 3: How Fasting Impacts Weight Loss

We have discussed the science and effects fasting has on your body, but let's take that information and apply it directly to weight loss. We have mentioned weight loss regarding fasting, but how is this put into practice? You cannot simply fast for a week and expect drastic weight loss. However, by keeping fasting a part of our everyday diet, we allow our body to adapt to changes more easily, and thus can implement other practices that go hand in hand with fasting to ensure maximum results. Remember, weight loss is not only attributed to calorie restriction, but definable results are also seen with overall physical and mental health. Let's start with why we want to lose weight in the first place.

Physical appearance plays an integral role in our society. Billboards and commercials fill the air with super skinny models, forcing our minds to think that there is one true way women are supposed to look. This is completely unfair, and it attacks the mind as a whole. In good practice, we should try and avoid these thought patterns as much as possible and focus on our personal goals. Physically appearing attractive does not imply health. Too skinny, too fat – these words mean nothing if our bodies and minds are not balanced and healthy. So, let's find out why we want to cut weight with a few personal questions to ask ourselves: *Do I simply want to be beautiful? Do I want to lose weight for longevity? Is my body shape hindering me in some way? Do I need to lose weight for health purposes?* Even the healthiest of people will strive for more balance. No attainable end goal applies to everyone. You need to find your ideal goal and go from there. By taking time to contemplate why we want to or need to lose weight, we can hone in on our specific goals and aspire to attain them through specific practices directed at specific results.

Once we find ourselves being truthful with ourselves about body image, we can begin a true weight loss practice and with it a fasting regimen. But how will this fasting help us cut weight? Aside from the science showing us that Intermittent Fasting reduces inflammation, assists in hormone regulation, and burns cleaner energy, we need to view the fast through a psychological lens.

By even thinking about starting an IF routine, you have already started to change your life. The thoughts that cross your mind about wanting something better for yourself is just the beginning of what could become a dramatic life-altering transformation. The desire for longevity and to be healthful are very common goals; unfortunately, many people suppress these desires in exchange for an easier, way less healthy lifestyle. As this downward spiral progresses, one becomes caught in a seemingly endless loop of processed foods, social media, and laziness. By digging ourselves out of the typical routine, we have the opportunity to reinvent ourselves, to break the wicked cycle, and begin a new life. IF is a great place to begin for this process – not only do you break the detrimental meal cycle, but you also begin to see changes in your thought processes about everything else in your life that may be preventing you from living a healthy and happy life. By being persistent and dedicated, we can begin breaking away from the standard lifestyle. By eliminating the unneeded stress, we also assist ourselves in losing our unneeded weight.

The relationship between stress and obesity has been studied extensively, and there is a link between the two. As the obesity rate began to increase quickly in the United States, scientists soon realized that the problem wasn't limited to only wealthy countries but was a global problem. Thought initially to be a product of overeating and lack of exercise, soon studies showed that many other factors contributed to this pressing issue. Obesity-related illnesses have been linked to industrial, cultural, and, of course, genetic predispositions –all being stressors that are out of our control. Our surroundings cause these stressors, and our society plays a huge role in weight management. Stress is a response in our bodies that is critical for survival. The 'flight or fight' response ensured our survival in prehistoric times and allowed us to adapt to our environment. When we are stressed, our autonomic nervous system is activated; this system regulates heart rate, blood pressure, hormone regulation, and digestion. As we see here, these are the same major functions that IF has been shown to help balance and regulate.

Many of the people who have problems with obesity react to stress by eating food. However, this 'comfort' food is not worth the trouble. Much of the comforting food is very high in fats and sugar, not to mention usually consumed outside of the individual's routine. This may serve as a quick fix for stress, but it can lead to addiction-like behavior and overeating. It is no secret that the food that is valued in our culture is not very healthy, and with the advent of GMO foods and soil that is depleted of nutrients from pesticides, even our fruits and vegetable are not up to par. The food problem is a huge issue today, in fact, unavoidable, but there are ways we go about our lives that counteract much of the problem. Eating nutrient-rich foods that are grown locally and avoiding frozen or prepackaged meals will go a long way to reduce stress. We will go into detail about the suitable meals for IF in a later chapter. By being mindful about our relationship with food is only going to help us in our journey to transformation.

Another issue with weight loss is physical activity. Many people feel that they do not have time to exercise or simply have become so out of shape that the idea of exercise never comes to mind: this is unacceptable. Some may hear the word exercise and instantly picture in their minds a sweaty, beefed-up man lifting weights in front of a mirror. This is a very narrow-minded approach to exercise. Instead of these stereotypical ideas of what it takes to be healthy, let's consider less intensive images. Someone in normal everyday clothing walking casually on a trail in the wilderness or perhaps slowly stretching on a yoga mat in a quiet room – this is exercise too. We don't have to hit the gym to have a balanced physical lifestyle, but simply moving around and getting the blood flowing can suffice. Studies have shown that stress is reduced with a casual exercise routine that even in the moments of the stressful situation, a quick stretch or walk around the block will help alleviate the stress. We will discuss the relationship between IF and exercise later.

So, we see that stress is an important aspect of weight management; it affects the very same major functions that IF has been shown to affect. Combined with a more mindful diet, moderate exercise, and truthful self-image, we see the formation of a very safe and effective routine for weight loss. Now, let's look at what is happening to excess fat when we are in the midst of a fast.

As discussed above, we have found that fasting improves health in many ways. The most accepted science on IF states that fasting influences the circadian rhythms and various other systems needed to live. Circadian rhythms are built in biological processes that act like a biological clock, similar to other natural rhythms such as the tides or seasonal rhythms. These rhythms are controlled by the hypothalamus and can be altered and trained from outside influences, such as light, darkness, food, and IF, respectfully. Organs in your body respond to food restriction and can act to reset these rhythms. Food restriction also affects the microbiome of your gut – all the bacteria and ecosystem of your gut has its own rhythm as well. As your body resets and the energy from your latest meal is used up, the body turns to fat reserves. The fat reserves release fatty acids which find their way to the liver where they are then converted into ketones. The ketones provide energy for muscles and help to prevent disease processes by protecting neurons. Although, if ketone levels become too high, it could be dangerous. This complicated process is the underlying physical benefit of IF: resetting the internal clocks and using fat reserves. The fat reserves having been reduced, we now find ourselves weighing less safely and effectively. When considering this, we need to dig a little deeper into what ketosis is and how it works.

Ketosis

Much information you find online about IF or weight loss leads to websites and articles dedicated to ketosis and keto diets. Although the ketosis diets are not mandatory for IF, it is a good idea to be educated on the process of ketosis itself and how it interplays with IF.

Ketosis pops up a lot in conversations about health and current diet trends; it is one of the more popular diets on the Internet and yields plenty of success stories from people who practice the diet. But what is ketosis exactly? It can be a positive or a negative thing depending on the context and situation. Ketosis is a natural process that occurs in the body as a metabolic process. Similar to what we've discussed, when your body doesn't have any quick energy to burn, such as carbohydrates from a recent meal, it will burn stored fat instead. This process makes ketones. If the ketone levels in the blood get too high, there can be complicated problems – typically insulin and other hormones prevent the ketone levels from getting too high. However, if there are issues with insulin production, this can be an issue. This is why people with diabetes find themselves in an unwanted ketosis state if they're not using enough insulin and often avoid inducing the state intentionally. A healthy normal body that consumes a balanced diet is in control of the amount of fat it burns and typically won't make ketones. Aside from just restricting carbohydrate intake, ketosis can also be induced by pregnancy and long exercise routines. The ketosis state can most certainly be viewed as a survival mechanism built into the human body. When we have no quick energy to use, or we have no food to ingest, our body switches over to creating ketones and using stored fat to power the body. We see here how ketosis fits into our IF lifestyle. If we restrict calories, especially from carbohydrate-rich foods, the ketosis state will take hold, and we can start burning unwanted and excess fat.

As a weight loss strategy, ketosis diets are effective and safe when practiced with attention to our bodies and state of mind. Not unlike a paleo diet or the popular Atkins diet from decades ago, the low-carb strategy can be very beneficial if used wisely. The diet has been shown to assist the body to maintain muscle and make you feel less hungry. Obviously, fasting will induce a ketosis-like state very quickly, but reducing carbohydrate intake to less than 60 grams a day for four to five days can start a ketosis-like state as well. The diet has been implemented to some success for treatment of many serious diseases including epilepsy.

As with any diet, a ketogenic diet needs to be practiced with great care and with meticulous attention to your body's changes. If the ketone levels in your body get too high, they can build up in the blood and ketoacidosis can take hold. Ketoacidosis causes the built-up ketones to turn the blood very acidic and can result in a coma or even death. Ketone levels can be tested in urine or blood, and it is always a good idea to test if you choose to practice a ketogenic diet. Along with unsafe fasting practices, ketoacidosis can be caused by alcoholism, dehydration, and an overactive thyroid. If you are affected by these symptoms, it is best to check with your doctor before attempting any diet or fast that may induce a ketogenic state.

So, not only do we see an IF routine as directly affecting our circadian rhythms and reducing fat, but the practice acts as a building block to other weight loss protocol. Through fasting, we influence the systems of the body that cause stress, while simultaneously taking societal stress off ourselves by developing a better diet and attitude. The IF routine affects our idea of exercise, not only by freeing time to exercise but also by inducing a ketosis-like state and exercising. We burn fat reserves quicker than if we were eating the same foods at the same time. This combination will be the basis of our weight loss regimen. Now, we need to find a fasting technique that is best suited to our needs.

As we continue on our transformative journey, with science in mind, we need to explore the many different ways we can introduce IF into our lives. There is an infinite number of ways to start your IF routine, but we will focus on some of the more prominent methods that have taken the Internet by storm in recent years.

Chapter 4: Different Intermittent Fasting Techniques

Now that we have discussed how your body will react to fasting let's discuss the many different forms of fasting. Although there are seemingly infinite ways to go about your Intermittent Fasting routine, we will focus on six methods that are popular among fitness experts and the fasting community. We will discuss the suitable timing of 'eating windows', the duration of time in the day when you are allowed to eat, and compare each method so you can successfully choose the best one for your lifestyle. Although fasting has its roots in religion and spirituality, we will not go extensively into these practices, but if you wish to combine your spiritual goals with these methods, you can go right ahead.

At this point, we would like to state that keeping a fasting notebook helps immensely for someone just starting out. By recording our experiences and documenting how successful or unsuccessful our routine is, we can find insight into ourselves and also organize the aspects of our routine that may need to be altered or customized. It is not mandatory to have a notebook, but throughout this book, we will be keeping track of our experiences and analyzing our regimen to understand better what works for us as individuals.

As we move on to explore these popular methods, take note of what they entail and which styles pique your interest as you learn about them. The methods we will explore are as follows:

1. The 16/8 Method
2. The 5:2 Method
3. The Eat Stop Eat Method
4. Alternating Day Fasts
5. The Warrior Method
6. The Spontaneity Method

We will also be discussing tips for customizing your routine. The point of this is to personalize your fasting, so it suits you perfectly. This will optimize the results and also allow the practice to become something you created for yourself, which in turn, builds an intimate relationship with your practice promoting dedication and confidence.

The particular method you choose will have a great deal to do with your day-to-day schedule and mindset. Let's choose wisely and give much thought to the various benefits of different methods, but keep in mind the result can be obtained through any of these methods. Let's also be fair in saying that the time windows can be altered to give or take an hour if need be. If one method doesn't quite work for you, do not be disheartened; simply try another method or customize your current choice.

The 16/8 Method

Also known as the Leangain's method, this method was popularized by Martin Berkhan. The eating window for this style is eight hours with a sixteen-hour fasting time. So if you sleep eight hours, awake, then restrict caloric intake for eight hours, then you can eat as much as you like until bedtime. Another example would be to awake, start your eight-hour eating window, then begin fasting for the evening and during sleep. This is a common choice for people who already skip breakfast. Tea and coffee have no calories, so they are still allowed to be consumed, obviously without sugar added.

Overview:
- Sixteen hours of fasting
- Eight-hour consumption window
- Zero-calorie drinks allowed

The 5/2 Diet Method

This method looks more like a diet than a proper fast, but it is a popular method for weight loss and often finds its way into IF circles. First popularized by Michael Mosley, it is also called the 'Fast Diet'. This method involves your normal eating routine for five days of the week then restricting your caloric intake to 600 calories or less for two days of the week. So you can choose your two days to fast whether they are together or not, let's say Wednesday and Friday. Then, treat all other days as normal days, but on Wednesday and Friday, you eat one or two small meals that together equal 600 calories or less. This is a great beginner diet to try before you get into some more intensive IF. If you're wary of how you may react to fasting, then this method is great to start.

Overview:
- Five days of normal meals according to your daily diet
- Two days of consuming 600 calories or less

The Eat Stop Eat Method

This method was popularized by Brad Pilon and involves a strict 24-hour fast one to two times a week. That is 24 hours of no solid food or caloric intake. Unsweetened coffee and tea are acceptable during the fasting days for this method. A great example would be to fast from dinner to dinner or, let's say, from 4:00 pm to 4:00 pm the next day. It does not matter what time frame you choose, but it should be a solid 24-hour period. Keeping to your usual eating schedule on the non-fasting days is important.

Overview:
- Strict 24-hour fast once or twice a week
- Maintain usual eating schedule during non-fast days

The Alternating Day Method

This method involves fasting every other day. This method can be customized to your liking on the fast days. You can cut back to 600 calories a day, not unlike the 5/2 method, but fasting every other day. If you feel comfortable, you can intake zero calories on the fast days; this would be a very intense method and is not recommended for beginners. For example, eat normally on Sunday, lower calorie intake to 600 calories or less on Monday, eat normally on Tuesday, lower calorie intake Wednesday, eat normally on Thursday, lower calories on Friday. You see, we hit a snag in our pattern as there is an odd number of days in a week. For the odd day out, in this case, Saturday, you can choose to lower the calorie count or eat regularly. It is up to you. For another example, the Saturday odd day out, you could potentially fast for 24 hours then jump back into the pattern on Sunday.

Overview:
- Fast or lower calories every other day
- Keep a usual eating schedule on non-fast days
- Choose what suits you best for the odd day out

The Warrior Method

This method was popularized by Ori Hofmekler. It includes eating small amounts of raw plant-based foods during the day, then one large meal during the evening. Essentially, you are fasting all day and breaking the fast at night. This diet typically focuses on eating raw and unprocessed foods to get the full benefit. For example, during the day, you snack on fruits, veggies, and nuts. Once the evening comes, you prepare a large meal that is as unprocessed and raw as possible.

Overview:
- Light amounts of raw foods or completely fasting during daylight hours
- A large meal at night, as unprocessed and raw as possible

The Spontaneity Method

This method is the loosest and most flexible method of IF. The method is pretty straight forward; there are no guidelines or structures. Simply skip a meal when it's convenient or if you're not hungry. Skipping one or two meals every so often can be a great foundation to lay while you search for a more suitable routine. This method also comes in handy for busy people, parents, or just people who love winging it.

Overview:
- No structure
- Simply skip meals when convenient, or fast whenever you like

Customization Techniques

Now that we have a general idea of different fasting techniques let's keep in mind that these are guidelines that can be customized to fit your specific lifestyle. To reiterate: no one way suits everyone. So as you analyze these methods, keep in mind your personal life and how you alter the structures not only to fit into your schedule but also to personalize your practice. By personalizing your routine, you allow yourself some added empowerment and something that you helped create. Some examples of customizing your practice can include changing the length of fasts, changing diet to suit (vegan, Paleo, etc.), and/or changing the fasting patterns (alternating every two days, etc.).

With the methods above, we see many similarities between them. With the main premise being a caloric restriction and eating window restriction, these methods are simply different customized versions of fasting itself. So this means that we can customize these methods to suit our needs and preferences as individuals.

When we decide to customize a method, it needs to be well thought out. *Why do I need these customizations? Are these customizations feasible as something I can accomplish?* There is an infinite number of ways we can change and alter these techniques, and we will provide some examples below. Keep in mind these are not the only ways to customize but just some basic strategies. Customize as you please, but be safe and mindful in doing so:

- **Customization Strategy #1**: Altering the duration of eating windows

We see above that one of the main differences in these methods is the timing. For example, the 16/8 method requires eating for eight hours of the day and fasting for sixteen hours of the day. This can be altered easily to suit you. Need a little extra time for the eating window? Add an hour. Feeling confident that you can shorten the eating window? Shorten it an hour or two. You can also choose your eating window during the day. Morning, midday, or night are all suitable times to eat depending on your schedule.

- **Customization Strategy #2**: Altering days

The days in which you choose to fast are very important but not limited to the guidelines above. The alternating method as an example, alternating days of fasting is a simple pattern, but what if you need two days off from fasting? Make your fast days every third day. Another example would be putting more fast days together, as with the Eat Stop Eat method. Instead of one or two days of complete calorie restriction, maybe do three or push your two days back-to-back for a more challenging fast.

- **Customization Strategy #3**: Altering the timing of meals

Much content online will suggest a proper time for having your meals or will cite the warrior method as an example that requires a large meal at night. This large meal can be placed anywhere in the day according to your preference; in fact, many people prefer their large meal in the middle of the day to avoid a full stomach while sleeping.

- **Customization strategy #4**: Altering meal choices

As noted above, the warrior method requires raw foods to be ingested. Many people have dietary restrictions and preferences that may not fit into these diets and methods, so switch it up! What you eat during your IF routines is important, and you want to keep it healthy. But be reasonable with yourself; choose foods you enjoy. If you prefer fried, greasy foods, maybe try the same ingredients but prepared differently – baked chicken instead of breaded and fried, etc.

- **Customization strategy #5**: Include your lifestyle

When we research fasting online, we see a pattern – health blogs with muscular people in their fitness attire smiling brightly in front of a sunset. This is all fine for some people, but many do not relate to this lifestyle. Lucky for us, fasting is for everyone. You can add fasting to your normal routine easily without hitting the gym or buying spandex. Make it a point to meld IF into your lifestyle rather than view it as something separate from you. Any hobby you love – gaming, fishing, reading, music, art, scrapbooking, etc. – can be a part of your fasting routine. In fact, having a low-intensity hobby is great for the downtime during fasts. Let's not be discouraged if you're not a health nut. Include fasting regardless of your preferred lifestyle, and it will improve it.

These five strategies barely scratch the surface of all the different ways we can alter our routine to fit our lifestyles. Often enough, when we start a fasting routine and get comfortable with the practice, it alters itself naturally to suit our lives. Move with the natural current of things and let your body do the talking. Think deeply on the many strategies available to you and find creative ones to personalize your practice.

We've examined some of the more popular methods of IF and how any method can be altered and customized to fit anyone's needs. While the methods listed above are not the end-all-be-all of IF, they are some of the more popular techniques for a reason. The fitness experts and health gurus that meticulously study and practice these methods present them for the masses online because they work. Another factor being that in our fast-paced society, these methods seem to be some of the better fitting techniques.

Along with promoting these practices, we find much debate online about the validity of fasting and its benefits for the body. Let's explore some common myths and misconceptions.

Chapter 5: Fasting and Exercise Myths Explained

As the popularity of Intermittent Fasting grows, many voices can be heard speaking negatively about the practice. This is understandable as fasting is a taboo in the Western-developed world, seemingly depriving oneself of necessary nutrition would frighten anyone with a conscience. Fears pertaining to exercise are very common. It would seem that not having any food intake would make exercise out of the question, but it will depend on the type of exercise and, of course, your overall health. It is very important to read this section thoroughly, so you don't contradict the work you've done to better yourself. Many myths can be found online, but let's analyze these allegations and apply the science we've learned to debunk any fears and ensure the safest and most effective means of exercise while Intermittent Fasting.

We've seen the science of this kind of fasting allowing our body to use our fat reserves for a cleaner and more efficient energy, but is exercise going to disrupt this process? And if not, what exercises are the most useful? Here we will discuss an IF and exercise combination, while also debunking some other myths pertaining to exercising on an empty stomach.

Let's start with some basic misconceptions about fasting:

Intermittent Fasting Will Slow Your Metabolism

This is a very misunderstood concept. While you fast, your body is going to try to compensate for the disrupted meal routine, but your metabolic rate will not slow; it will simply go about its business as usual. If your body were somehow to use up all its energy and fat reserves, then you would be considered to be 'undereating', and this is when the metabolism slows, and you could be in potential harm's way. So, instead of focusing solely on the idea that fasting is calorie restriction, view it as more of a restriction of the time when you're allowed to intake calories.

By Just Fasting You Will Lose Weight

As we have discussed, losing weight isn't going to happen overnight just because you restrict calories. Developing a nutrient-rich diet alongside casual exercise with IF fasting will be much more effective. Eating pizza every chance you get is not a mindful approach to fasting or a balanced diet, which leads us to the next myth.

You Can Eat Anything You Want In Between Fasts

Ending a fast then diving into a processed food coma is about as counterproductive as it gets. Maintaining healthy eating habits outside of fasting days is going to be a very important key to losing weight and keeping it off. Try to avoid using your fasting practice as an excuse to overindulge.

Intermittent Fasting Is Effective and Everyone Sees Results

This has been a big one throughout the book. No one practice is going to suit everyone. Each individual is very different. Although we all share a basic structure, genes and environment play a huge role in what practices work and what doesn't. Let's not be discouraged though; we can customize our practice and find what works best with just a little time and effort.

Fasting Is Starving Yourself and Unhealthy

We've touched on this one, and it is very common. You express to a peer that you're going to start fasting and they are taken aback by your statement. They think you're going to get hurt or starve to death, and this just isn't true. We've discussed the science, and if used correctly, these ancient practices are safe. Let us keep in mind that we are transforming ourselves through fasting; we are using it as a structure and foundation to a healthy and happy life.

Fasting Leads to Muscle Loss

This is a popular argument for people who oppose fasting. However, the truth is that muscles that are used on a regular basis and plenty of protein ensure the muscle's health. In fact, if the body is searching for fuel, it is not likely to go after muscle since stored fat is way more efficient. Keep in mind, though, that you do not have unlimited fat reserves.

Now, for some myths regarding exercise in general, there is much debate among scientists and people all around the world about what counts as proper exercise and which workouts and regimens are the best. We will continue on our path of 'Everyone is individual and requires customized fitness' as we explore these common misconceptions.

Exercising Leads to Weight Loss

Yes, you need exercise to stay fit, but exercise alone will not suffice. Do not assume that if you eat a pizza, you can simply go 'run it off'. Most studies show that to lose weight, you need balanced eating habits and regular exercise. In fact, many agree that a balanced diet plays an even bigger role in weight loss than the exercise itself.

The Best Time to Exercise Is in the Morning

Exercising in the morning is a popular routine that many people adhere to, but this doesn't mean that it's the best time. Some studies show that exercise in the morning may help prime the body for fat burning during the day, but that's no reason to force a workout in the morning. The best time to exercise is when you feel is the best time. If you like late night runs, go for it. Do what you feel happy doing and make sure to keep active regularly.

Exercise Benefits Only the Physical

Another misconception is that the brain cannot be 'worked out' through exercise. This is untrue. Although puzzles and games help the brain, aerobic exercise seems to be the key to keeping your brain in shape.

Fasted Workouts

With these myths in mind, let's move on to some science about the combination of fasting and exercise or 'fasted workouts'. These workouts are very popular for morning fasts since you can wake up with a relatively empty stomach, have some water, and hit your workout. However, there is much controversy on the subject of exercise on an empty stomach. There are not many studies available on the practice specifically, so the debate continues. Whether or not you think it works better than exercise on a half-full stomach or not, this book is here to give you suitable information to make your own informed decisions.

So, we know that when the stomach is empty, and the body has no immediate access to energy, then it will rely on stored fats. This fact alone implies that working out during a fast would successfully burn unneeded fat reserves, thus leading to weight loss. Although weight loss is the main focus here, we also need to address the many other benefits that IF has when combined with exercise. Studies have shown that fasted cycling to enhance endurance was easier to recover from than endurance cycling with food in the stomach. Along with recovery from endurance exercises, we have seen an improved recovery from the wear and tear of weight training, so we see a pattern of improved recovery after a workout if the athlete was in a fasted state. Similarly, fasted workouts should have higher glycogen storage. By keeping glycogen levels low during workouts, your body adapts to running on low glycogen. Thus, when you have food in your stomach, the body will use its energy more efficiently since it is trained to do so.

These ideas may not be the most amazing practices for a professional athlete, but for a regular person looking to shed a few pounds or develop a new lifestyle, the practices seem optimal.

But what about the many different types of exercise?

Most experts agree that exercise is safe to do while on an empty stomach, but are you getting the most out of your workout? As far as we can tell, the following conclusions can be found:

If your workout requires high levels of speed and power, you will benefit from having food in your stomach. This is due to the high amount of energy you will be burning in a short amount of time, so the energy that is available to be burned quickly is ideal for getting the most out of your workout.

For an empty stomach or fasted workout, the experts suggest cardio and aerobic workouts on all levels, whether it's tai chi or a jog through the park, or intensive yoga and deep stretching. These less intense workouts are ideal practices during a fast and will be the most effective for weight loss.

It is also understood that if you wish to start a fasted cardio routine, you should not have any serious health conditions like low blood pressure or other conditions that may cause dizziness or increase the risk of injury. The following tips are a great guideline for beginners:

1. Stay hydrated. Consume plenty of water.
2. Do not work out for longer than an hour
3. Choose moderate or low-intensity workouts
4. Listen to your body. If you experience discomfort, then take a breather

In the following chapters, we will reference 'light exercise'. This may be self-explanatory, but it will not hurt to suggest some exercise practices that pair well with IF. These exercises are light and not tough on the body, but we should still break a nice sweat when we are performing these 'light' exercises.

Some fitting ideas for fasted exercise:

- **Yoga**

    Sanskrit for 'union', this traditional Indian practice sets out to unite the body and mind by combining intricate poses and stretches with structured breathing exercises. Cultural influence aside, even spending ten to fifteen minutes a day dedicated to stretching the body and focusing some attention on deep breathing will do wonders as a warmup to a workout or a workout in and of itself.

    You can find plenty of books and online resources to find a yoga practice that suits you. The practice aims to strengthen the body while also furthering flexibility. It is a great core workout and really assists us in getting to know our body and its boundaries.

- **Tai Chi**

    As a traditional Chinese martial art, this practice is designed to teach the practitioner how to control and manipulate the subtle energies of the body and its surroundings. Somewhat similar to yoga, this practice involves the constant movement of postures rather than holding poses. Breath is just as important during tai chi as in yoga. As a general rule, being in control of your breathing is a key component to a mindful and healthy life.

There is an abundant amount of material on tai chi online, and many major cities have multiple tai chi instructors and classes that meet in groups or one-on-one. Finding a class that takes place in a natural or relaxing setting is ideal.

- **Jogging**

All of us are familiar with jogging. The casual running exercise aims to build endurance and stamina by running at a steady pace at moderate speeds. Early morning jogs are a great way to start the day and pair well with a fasted morning.

You can jog anywhere. Jog around the block of your neighborhood or visit a school track or a gym that has running space to change the scenery. There are many running groups online if you feel uncomfortable running alone.

- **Cardio**

Cardio workouts are defined as any workout that gets your heart rate up. Jogging can be considered cardio, but there are meticulously designed cardio workouts that aim to burn fat through different intensities. Many workouts ask that you have intervals of intense cardio followed immediately by rest than more intense cardio.

There are hundreds of different cardio styles and workouts available online to suit your skill level and lifestyle. Your local gym should have machines perfect for cardio and possibly even classes dedicated to weight loss through cardio. Cycling machines and the elliptical are popular machines you can find at gyms for cardio workouts.

- **Pilates**

Very similar to yoga, but with more strength building exercises, Pilates was invented in the twentieth century as an effective way to tone muscle without bulking up. It pairs well with IF since it is low impact and can be performed anywhere, not unlike yoga.

Most cities should have Pilates instructors nearby, and there are abundant resources online.

- **Hiking**

This is a low-impact, relaxing, and thought-provoking activity. Taking a hike in the woods is an immersive experience. There's something very beneficial about being in a natural setting away from all the hustle and bustle of a town or city. Depending on the terrain, hiking can be a casual stroll or close to a treacherous climb. The combination of fasting and hiking is an amazing one as you notice your senses are heightened as you walk empty-bellied through the forest.

There are hiking trails all around the world, and they often state the intensity level of the hike. Searching for new trails and scenic spots quickly becomes a hobby that is beneficial on many levels. Adventurous, educational, self-reflective, and most certainly great for your body, hiking is paired wonderfully with IF since you are in control of how difficult it is. But, of course, if you are fasting and going out into the woods, be sure to bring plenty of water and emergency snacks.

Chapter 6: Best Foods for Fasting

Moving forward, as we get ever closer to our goal of completely changing our outlook on the diet, we find ourselves with a bit of an appetite. But what foods are okay to eat while fasting? Although you could safely keep your normal diet and simply fast around it, we can optimize our transformation by including foods that are ideal to pair with a diet that includes regular Intermittent Fasting. With access to nearly any food we desire, it is tough not to grab the pizza slice or burger when we feel hungry. However, we're developing our confidence and control here, not simply fulfilling our immediate desires. By taking control of our instant desires, we empower ourselves to think mindfully of our next meal, and a dedicated IF regime assists us in accomplishing this life-altering goal.

First things first, let's take a moment to think about our diets. Go back one week and write out all the meals you had including snacks and contemplate it:

Were these foods I desired? Were these foods of convenience? Were there any foods that could have been easily left out? Were these foods rich in nutrients?

These questions are pretty straightforward, but let's try and be more abstract:

Where did the food come from? Was this food natural? What time of the day was I eating? Was it a set routine? Why did I choose these particular foods? Was this the same diet I've maintained for over a decade?

This contemplation should be thorough and invigorating. There will be realizations and even more questions, more intimate ones. Let the thought process flow over you. This is a beginning step to being mindful of your diet. These simple questions will help prepare you for how your diet will change once IF begins. You will consciously change your habits, but you will also subconsciously be building a relationship with your desires and changing them from the inside out. Keep your diet in mind leading up to the fast and consider some options below if they haven't been in your diet before.

Many fad diets come and go over the years, but in reality, they are just that – fads. Cutting out carbs or only eating protein isn't going to give us the well-rounded, transformative effect we're searching for here. We need to balance our diet, explore nutrient-rich ingredients, and find alternatives to the ingredients that are most detrimental to our goals.

Moving forward, let us investigate what type of diets are best suited for IF. Since it requires you only to eat during certain parts of the day or only on certain days, we need not to just stuff ourselves with whatever we get our hands on but to be mindful of how balanced our meals are. Since we aim to lose weight while simultaneously transforming the way we view meals and food, we need meals and snacks that are mostly unprocessed, high in fiber, and have lean protein. But what we eat isn't the only factor. If you think about a 'normal' day of eating, you will realize that our digestive system is working from morning until night to digest three or more meals a day. This is just asking for weight gain since our stomachs are never empty, and our body doesn't need to burn our fat reserves for energy. So, we soon realize that the time we eat is also important. The timing will be covered in subsequent chapters.

As we think about raw, nutrient-rich food, we also consider where our food comes from. Foods produced locally will be richer in nutrients and promote the local economy by supporting smaller farms. This is a practice in mindfulness as we seek to develop a better relationship with food and, through this mindful notion, contribute to a more ecologically and economically balanced world around us. Since we seek to better ourselves through transformation, our relationship with food needs to be reevaluated, and an excellent place to start is where your food is sourced. You will also learn more about the foods available to you, educating yourself on which foods are in the season, thus helping you decide what foods you will be preparing during fasting weeks. Taking a visit to your local farmer's market is more than likely the best option for sourcing local foods, not to mention the relationship you build with other people who share the same notion of community support.

Here are some foods that are rich in nutrients and are ideal for a fasting lifestyle:

Leafy Greens

Deep, dark, leafy greens are a staple in the optimized fasting diet. These foods are rich in vitamins A, C, and K as well as plenty of potassium and fiber. These greens can replace the standard lettuce in any recipe and are available all year round. Kale, among many other leafy greens, is even considered one of the most nutrient-rich foods known to humans. If you are not a fan of the flavor of leafy greens, blend them up in a smoothie with some fruits to mask the taste. Some examples of delicious leafy greens include kale, spinach, collard greens, chard, turnip greens, and cabbage.

Garlic

Garlic is found in many recipes and can be eaten raw if you don't mind the pungent flavor and aroma. High in B vitamins, vitamin C, calcium, copper, and selenium, this nutrient-rich food could potentially lower and balance blood pressure while also containing antibacterial and antifungal properties. Garlic can be a welcome ingredient in most meals, minced or whole.

Potatoes

Potatoes are versatile and fun to cook with. They pack a massive amount of potassium, copper, and iron while also containing a good amount of vitamins B and C. Another ideal factor for IF is how filling a potato can be. Try boiling potatoes for the most beneficial preparation method.

Tomatoes

With a wide variety of different types to choose from, tomatoes are versatile and yield many different flavors. Packed full of vitamins and minerals, these beautifully bright foods can be eaten raw by themselves or added to salads.

Broccoli

Notorious for being hated by many people, broccoli is full of vitamins C and K among other vitamins and minerals. Best steamed or eaten raw in salads.

Cauliflower

Cauliflower is an incredibly nutrient-rich food that deserves way more attention. Vitamin C, K, B12, and filled with fiber, this vegetable has much-needed minerals and small amounts of protein. Find creative recipes online or eat raw in salads.

Sunflower Seeds

An excellent source of vitamin E, these tiny seeds are great to snack on. Antioxidants, copper, phosphorous, and magnesium abound in these little seeds. Add to any salad or eat raw.

Almonds

Nuts and seeds are wonderful for snacking during IF. Almonds, in particular, pack a bunch of vitamin E, copper, magnesium, and fiber. One downside is the large number of calories, so be cautious while on a restricted caloric intake and snacking on almonds.

Blueberries

Among the many berries and their many benefits, blueberries stand out when it comes to being rich in nutrients. Although not as rich in vitamins as most vegetables, blueberries boast a wild amount of antioxidants, which can protect the brain and repair cells. Throw some blueberries in a salad or snack on them raw.

Raspberries

Although a little tough to find in some places, if you can get your hands on some raspberries, you can fulfill your body's needs for vitamin C, fiber, and manganese. Eat raw, with yogurt, or in smoothies.

Chocolate

You're probably thinking of name brands of candy bars right now, but in all seriousness, dark chocolate is packed with antioxidants, fiber, iron, magnesium, and copper. Grabbing chocolate with 80% or higher cocoa content is the healthiest. Mix it with smoothies, nuts, or eat raw.

Beans

Beans, black beans, in particular, are filled with iron and protein. They are filling and great to replace red meats for protein content that is much leaner. Plenty of minerals and folic acid come along with the versatile bean. Cook in chili, burritos, or even salads.

Rice

Among other whole grains, rice is rich in fiber and small amounts of vitamins and minerals. Rice is one of the most consumed foods in the world and can be mixed and paired with almost anything. Sweet or savory, rice goes a long way when fasting. It is filling, inexpensive, and easy to cook. Pair with sautéed vegetables, fish, tofu, and beans.

Tofu

Fermented soybean doesn't sound appealing to everyone, but tofu is incredibly versatile and is a great source of lean, plant-based protein. As a great alternative to red meats and other animal proteins, tofu is a lynchpin in a vegetarian or vegan diet. Marinate and sauté with veggies or press and fry for sandwiches.

Salmon

Salmon stands out among fish as a nutrient-rich powerhouse. Filled with omega-3 fatty acids and plenty of protein, salmon also helps lower heart disease. Replace beef or other meats with salmon two to three times a week for a leaner, more nutrient-rich protein source.

Shellfish

Shellfish may be the most nutritious sea creatures we know of. Clams, oysters, and mussels, among others, rank high on the oceanic food list. Excellent sources of B12 and other vitamins, these foods also contain a ton of zinc, potassium, and iron. Consume sparingly perhaps on a celebratory night out or during other special occasions.

The foods mentioned above are some of the highest valued foods for IF. Work them into your diet as well as you can, and don't be afraid to get creative with preparation techniques. Keep note of the foods that you already have in your diet and the ones you want to add to your new diet.

Meal Prepping

Along with developing a balanced and fast-friendly diet, there are techniques to take the complicated process of preparing and cooking every meal. Meal prepping, or simply meal prep, is an excellent way to save time during busy weeks, especially if you are implementing your new IF regimen. This technique is pretty straightforward: prepare all your meals for a week and store them in a container until they are ready to use. As simple as this is, let's go over some steps that often get overlooked to get you started. We will keep this step-by-step list focused on IF for the sake of our goals.

Step #1: Decide what food you want to prep

Make a list of mostly raw or unprocessed foods that you wish to consume throughout the upcoming week. Are you having the same meal every day? Or are you switching it up day to day? Once you decide what you wish to prep, head to the grocery store and be sure to buy plenty for a week's worth of meals. Some people like to choose a calorie limit and choose meals that stay under a certain caloric intake per meal. Once you have the meals in mind, continue on.

Step#2: Choose a day to prep

Your refrigerator is stocked, and you're ready to prep. Find out when your fast begins and prepare the food the day before you start. This way, the food will stay fresh longer into your week-long fast.

Step#3: Obtain containers

You will need containers to keep your prepared meals in. Tupperware and the other storage ware you have available will suffice, but many buy containers that have divided sections for the different foods. The containers need to be airtight and BPA-free. Here's a short list of features your containers should have:

- BPA-free
- Reusable
- Microwave safe
- Stackable

Once you have your containers, you can start preparing the food.

Step#4: Prepare food

It's the day before you start your fast, so take your chosen ingredients and prepare them as you wish. Divide the foods out in seven equal parts for each day of the week, and then put them in the containers and store in the refrigerator. Keep in mind that uncooked foods will keep fresh longer and also pick things that will not require any further cooking or preparation once it's time to eat. Of course, having to reheat sometimes is necessary.

Step#5: Begin your week

You have your meals ready to go, and you don't need to worry about what to eat for a whole seven days. It's a nice relief – just don't forget to bring your prepared meal with you if you leave the house!

Meal prepping is a great way to keep control of your calorie intake and organize a new IF routine. With such a structured technique, it's nearly impossible to slip up on your goals. The steps above are a great foundation for an IF week. Alter the steps and quantities as you need to according to your fasting guidelines.

Below we will recommend some foods that are perfect for meal prep. Let's discuss the main courses and recommend some suitable examples of ingredients for these times of the day. The reference guide below will be focused on mostly raw unprocessed foods.

Breakfast

Breakfast is thought to be the most important meal of the day. However, this idea is flawed because it takes an entire balanced day of food to create a healthful life. No one meal is any important than the other; they all work together to create health and fulfillment. For our purposes in this book, we want breakfast foods that will not bog us down, so avoiding meats, bread, and sugary foods is ideal. With these things in mind let's take a look at some nutrient-rich foods that are great for starting the day:

- **Fruits:** Yes, we're avoiding sweets, but the natural source of sugar in fruit is a world away from the refined sugars we find in breakfast cereals and processed milk. An apple on the go is simple and quick. Cutting some orange slices or melon the night before is a great way to have a quick bite in the morning. Fruits are fulfilling and bursting with flavor, so for an IF regimen they come in handy as a quick source of energy or a light snack for an empty stomach.

  To be clear, we are talking about raw fruits – not jellies or preserves, not an Apple Danish. Having fruit chopped and ready to eat in the refrigerator is a great habit to get into. A huge bowl of fruit salad is exceptionally tantalizing after a long fasting day.

  Preparation: raw, fruit salad, paired with peanut butter, smoothie

  Acceptable fruits: apples, watermelon, honeydew, cantaloupe, oranges, clementine, cherries, bananas (although bananas have the most sugar content)

- **Berries:** There are plenty of common misconceptions and confusion about whether or not berries are fruits. They technically are, but we'll give them a special section all to themselves. The protocol for berries is the same as fruit: have them raw or mixed in a salad.

Preparation: raw, dried, salad, paired with other fruits, smoothie

Acceptable berries: blackberry, strawberry, blueberry

- **Nuts and Seeds:** Like fruits, nuts and seeds make for a quick raw snack that can easily be taken on the go. When choosing nuts, be sure to pick ones that are not covered with sugar or flavors. So avoid chocolate-covered or honey-roasted versions. Sea-salted nuts and raw nuts are the best.

Preparation: raw or roasted, trail mix, paired with fruits, smoothie

Nutritious nuts: almonds, cashews, pistachios, pecans, pumpkin seeds, sunflower seeds, chia seed, hemp seed

- **Whole Grains:** There are many whole grains to choose from, and these grains offer a lot in the way of fiber and carious vitamins. It is wise to eat bread sparingly, but a nice whole grain slice will go a long way; perhaps even switch bread out for a lighter option like a tortilla. The versatility of rice is a lifesaver if you're on a budget.

Preparation: cooked into oatmeal, bread, rice dishes, paired with almost anything.

Nutritious whole grains: rice, corn, oats, quinoa

- **Water:** This is an obvious ingredient, but also just as the only thing you have in the morning, water is a great way to start the day. Just a couple of 8-oz glasses and you're good to go – no harm in skipping out on breakfast every once in a while.

- **Eggs:** With eggs in the morning, we're getting to some heavier, less ideal breakfast foods. For a leaner egg, avoid eating the yolk. But if you must have eggs and need something a little bit heavier, eggs offer a high-protein inexpensive kick-start to the day.

Preparation: soft boiled, egg white omelet with veggies

- **Honorable Mention – Black Coffee:** Although it's a surprise, coffee is actually very healthy for you, not to mention an awesome way to start the day with its complex flavors and caffeine content. Of course, for our purposes, we will not be adding sugar, syrups, or milk to our coffee. It is highly recommended to develop a palette for black coffee and buy yourself a coffee as organic and locally roasted as possible.

Breakfast is simple. It is not necessary to eat steak, eggs, and potatoes for breakfast to 'start your day right'. Give the body some time to ease into the day by staying light and rich in nutrients for your breakfast choices.

Lunch

Midday meals are important to those who work long days and need a much-needed break. This leads to many of us settling for fast foods and sandwiches that have little nutritional value. For those who are fasting much of the time, the first solid food intake of the day is during lunchtime, so the choices we make for this meal will influence greatly how our day turns out. Meal prepping and smoothies can save you from settling for less healthy and processed foods.

- **Fruits and Berries:** These two food groups are going to show up a lot, so let's get used to it. These sweet foods are great for those with a nagging sweet tooth, not to mention a great source of quick energy.
  Preparation: raw, dried, salad, paired with other fruits, smoothie
  Acceptable berries: blackberry, strawberry, blueberry
- **Vegetables:** With such a wide variety to choose from, there is a veggie for everyone. Rich in fiber and various vitamins, vegetables are an IF's best friend. We can chat all day about the variety of ways vegetables can be prepared and consumed, but for a midday meal, salad is King.

Preparation: steamed or sautéed, eaten raw or with salad
Nutritious vegetables: tomatoes, broccoli, Brussel sprouts, potatoes, kale, carrots, spinach, cauliflower

- **Nuts and Seeds:** Like fruits, nuts and seeds make for a quick raw snack that can easily be taken on the go. When choosing nuts, be sure to pick ones that are not covered with sugar or flavors. So avoid chocolate-covered or honey-roasted versions. Sea-salted nuts and raw nuts are the best.

Preparation: raw or roasted, trail mix, paired with fruits, smoothie
Nutritious nuts: almonds, cashews, pistachios, pecans, pumpkin seeds, sunflower Seeds, chia seed, hemp seed

- **Whole Grains:** There are many different whole grains to choose from, and these grains offer a lot in the way of fiber and carious vitamins. It is wise to eat breads sparingly, but a nice whole grain slice will go a long way perhaps even switch bread out for a lighter option like a tortilla. The versatility of rice is a lifesaver if you're on a budget.

Preparation: cooked into oatmeal, bread, rice dishes, paired with almost anything.
Nutritious whole grains: rice, corn, oats, quinoa

- **Chicken:** Very lean and readily available, chicken is carbohydrate free and has very little fat and calorie content. It is an easy transition to cut out red meats and replace them with chicken. It's easy to prepare and versatile.

Preparation: boiled, sautéed, not breaded, tossed in a salad
Nutritious chicken: Not breaded, lightly seasoned, free range

Dinner

The last full meal of the day, dinner/supper is typically reserved for heavy meals and entertaining guests. The evening meal sets the tone of the evening and often is the meal that is most well thought out throughout the day. Steaks, burgers, and other heavy entrées rule this meal in the Western world, but we want to find leaner and more nutritious options for our purposes.

- **Fish:** Eating fish in place of heavier, less lean meats is a great way to alter your evening diet for the fasting lifestyle. In place of steaks, burgers, and pork, substitute the more nutrient-rich and lighter variety of fish or seafood.

Nutritious fish: salmon, albacore, sardines, trout, oysters

Preparation: Cooked thoroughly, sautéed or steam

- **Chicken:** Very lean, and readily available, chicken is carbohydrate free and has very little fat and calorie content. It is an easy transition to cut out red meats and replace them with chicken. It's easy to prepare and versatile.

Preparation: boiled, sautéed, not breaded

Nutritious chicken: not breaded, lightly seasoned, free range

- **Tofu:** The go-to replacement for meat-based protein, tofu is a soybean product that is full of great protein. It is a staple in Eastern cultures, and the Western world is slowly getting on board. Tofu is almost flavorless by itself, but when marinated or combined with veggies in a rice dish, it's just as valuable as any meat.

- **Vegetables:** With such a wide variety to choose from, there is a veggie for everyone. Rich in fiber and various vitamins, vegetables are an IF's best friend. We can chat all day about the variety of ways vegetables can be prepared and consumed, but for an evening meal, a salad appetizer or a sautéed side dish are winners.

Preparation: steamed or sautéed

Nutritious vegetables: tomatoes, broccoli, Brussel sprouts, potatoes, kale, carrots, spinach, cauliflower

- **Whole Grains:** There are many different whole grains to choose from, and these grains offer a lot in the way of fiber and carious vitamins. It is wise to eat breads sparingly, but a nice whole grain slice will go a long way, perhaps even switch bread out for a lighter option like a tortilla. The versatility of rice is a lifesaver if you're on a budget.

Preparation: cooked into oatmeal, bread, rice dishes, paired with almost anything

Nutritious whole grains: rice, corn, oats, quinoa

This basic guide to what foods are best at which part of the day is great for developing your own diet plan.

Snacks

Light snacks throughout the day help to appease your appetite and offer a much-needed break from monotonous days. Keeping snack foods handy is also a practice and also for safety – just in case your fasting days get the best of you, and you find yourself losing all your energy. Although it's popular to keep processed snacks nearby, chips, candies, and sodas are not ideal or our goals at hand.

Preparation: raw, trail mix, organic prepackaged

Nutritious snacks: nuts, seeds, fruits, veggies, granola, dark chocolate

Notable Diets

With weight loss in mind, we should explore some popular diets that pair quite well with IF. There are a few diets that have hit the mainstream and come equipped with the guidelines and structure needed to optimize weight loss when paired with IF. While diets have served as the stand-in for what it takes to be healthy in recent decades, studies have shown that simply altering what foods you eat will not lead to a healthful and balanced life. Many subtle changes need to be implemented to achieve these goals. Yes, the food you eat is very important, but it's not the end-all-be-all of healthful practices. Going on a diet for a month doesn't change your life. If you want a healthy life and wish to maintain that health, you will need to balance all aspects of health – not just the food you eat. Below we will explore some diets and how they are perfect for IF.

Mediterranean Diet

This diet is inspired by the foods and nutritional outlook of people living near the Mediterranean Sea. Fruits, legumes, vegetables, and other plant-based foods rule this diet, along with an abundant amount of extra-virgin olive oil and fresh fish.

As it is well known, the culture and societies surrounding the Mediterranean are joyous about their meals, not to mention red wines. The celebratory nature of their lifestyles is no doubt key in their health and happiness. This mindful attitude is exactly what we aim for when it comes to our own relationships with food. The positive mindset, vegetables, fresh lean protein, and plenty of healthy fats make this diet, as well as the cultures that influence it, ideal for IF.

Paleo Diet

The Paleo diet, or caveman diet, is one of the more popular diets that has seen its fifteen minutes of fame but has continued onward after its initial boom in the mainstream media. The diet is loosely based on what we think our ancient ancestors consumed before agriculture and farming was developed. As far as studies go, it is thought that our ancestors were extremely active and ate a diet of organic and wild meats, nuts, greens, and even insects.

Many assume that the prehistoric man thrived mainly on meat, but this is a common misconception. Hunting alone would not yield enough food for a large tribe, so it's commonly thought that less than half of the diet would consist of meat. The rest of the diet would be filled with foraged foods like plants, berries, seeds, and nuts. Considering different regions around the world and the vague nature of studying the past, there is a lot of difference in opinion when it comes to the Paleo diet. It is safe to say that not all hunts would be successful, so there would be prolonged instances of sustaining on nothing but plant-based foods. This pattern of eating, in essence, is

IF. So the Paleo diet has a history with IF, but how can we apply this to the modern world?

There is no one strict structure for the Paleo diet. And given the variety of diets in the ancient world, on a scale from low-carb, high animal content to high-carb plant-based, many different styles can be considered 'paleo'. So, here is a general outline for what foods to eat with a basic Paleo diet:

- Meat (fish, lamb, beef, chicken, seafood)
- Eggs (free range, cage free)
- Vegetables (potatoes, broccoli, carrots, tomatoes)
- Nuts and Seeds (almonds, walnuts, sunflower seeds, pumpkin seeds)
- Fruits (apples, pears, oranges, avocados)
- Healthy Oils (extra virgin olive oil, coconut oil)
- Herbs (sea salt, rosemary, turmeric, garlic)

This list is a great stepping stone to more specific guidelines, and keep in mind this food should be as organic as possible, and the fruits, nuts, and herbs being wild foraged, of course. For a stricter regimen, here is a list of foods to avoid:

- Legumes (beans, lentils, peanuts)
- Grains (bread, pasta, wheat, rye, barley)
- Dairy (some diets allow butter and cheese)
- Some oils (soybean, corn, sunflower, grapeseed)
- Artificial sweeteners (sucralose, aspartame)
- Very processed foods (frozen, prepackaged, additives)

Ketogenic Diets

As we discussed briefly, ketosis is when your body has used up all its quick energy and creates ketones to help burn stored fat. Typically, these diets are all about high-fat, low-carbohydrate meals, like plenty of eggs, avocados, and fatty meats, while avoiding bread and whole grains which are the prime source of carbs in the contemporary diet.

By cutting back our carbohydrate consumption to 60 grams or less per day for four to five days, our body will begin to produce ketones, which allow the body to use stored fat. The body cannot directly use the fat on its own. This diet, paired with an IF routine, can be very effective for our weight loss purposes. However, we need to take into account the dangers that ketosis can be present for certain people. Avoid inducing ketosis if you have diabetes, are taking high blood pressure medication, or breastfeeding.

Vegetarian Diets

Vegetarian diets are popular all around the world and in many countries and cultures. Even within the scope of the Paleo diet, vegetarianism is acceptable at times. The diet is not only a healthy alternative to contemporary Western diets but is also more ecologically friendly compared to a diet where all the protein comes from animal-based sources. Many vegetarians choose this diet for the health benefits and their overall wellbeing, but many people find themselves practicing this diet for their love of animals and the earth.

As you are more than likely aware, the vegetarian's diet has a strict no-meat rule. This means no beef, pork, fish, chicken, or any other meat. Many vegetarians still consume eggs, eat butter, and use milk, but strictly no meat itself is consumed. Much of the scientific motivation behind the vegetarian diet is that plant-based proteins are better for you and easier to digest than red meats. Although this diet is just as balanced as any other, when approaching a vegetarian diet, it is important that you eat plenty of protein to make up for the immense amount of protein lost when cutting out meats. Another issue is iron and sodium intake that is found abundantly in meat. These building blocks of life need extra attention with a vegetarian diet. Regardless of motivation, the vegetarian diet is great for IF, with all the nutrient-rich ingredients found in the world of animal-free sustenance.

Vegan Diet

Another animal-free diet, the vegan diet is similar to the vegetarian diet, but instead of simply cutting out meat itself, this diet requires that you cut out all animal products. Eggs, milk, butter, and anything with the slightest bit of animal-related ingredients are off limits. This an extreme version of vegetarianism and even crosses over into other territories besides the individual's diet. Many vegans take pride in their decision to avoid all animal products every moment of their lives – no fur clothing, no products tested on animals, absolutely nothing that uses animals. This diet comes with a philosophy, and here in this book, our goals are elsewhere. There is plenty of information online about veganism.

The Whole30 Diet

This diet has seen a surge in popularity in recent years with the 'gluten-free' trend that has been going around. The diet itself calls for us to eliminate foods that are common culprits when it comes to allergies and intolerances. So it means cutting out gluten-rich grains and legumes like beans and peanuts. The diet involves a 30-day 'clean eating' cycle where you cut these potentially unhealthy foods out of your diet for 30 days, then see how you feel. You can gradually reintroduce these foods and again take note of your body's reactions. This diet can almost allow us to see if we are intolerant to certain foods, thus allowing us to cut out troublesome ingredients. This is also a great diet for developing mindfulness and awareness about our bodies. It will pair well with an IF week at the end of the 30-day cycle.

Raw Food Diet

The raw food diet is very similar to the vegan diet, and many vegans adhere to its basic principle of eating foods in their natural form. It includes raw fruits, vegetables, nuts, and seeds. Uncooked and not dehydrated or seasoned, the nutritional value of these foods in this diet cannot be debated. This diet is a pretty simple one, but it is more than likely a world away from your current diet. Some may find it difficult not to cook, and without cooking your meal choices are limited. This diet will be one of the more difficult to uphold, not to mention one of the more difficult diets to practice and also ensure that you get all the needed nutrients. However, if you feel like the raw food diet suits you, try it out and pay very close attention to what your body says in return.

With the incredible variety of diets available online, there's no shortage of plans, routines, and fads. It is best to avoid choosing a diet based on popularity and choose diets that you will actually enjoy. There's no reason to take all the joy out of eating and the art of cooking in exchange for a routine that may not even be very effective. With this in mind, we can safely say that if you find that a diet needs a little customization to suit your needs, then go ahead and alter it. This is your practice; this is your life. Take control and empower yourself regardless of what people say. Enjoyment of food and your lifestyle choices are just as important as the choices themselves. If we are not taking pleasure out of our choices, then we need to rearrange and alter our current routine.

Once we have established our preferred dietary choices or altered our diet to one with foods that are more suitable for IF, we can begin making preparations to start our fasting week.

Chapter 7: Getting Started

So, we've made it. We stand now with enough valuable information and proper preparation for setting a date to start including Intermittent Fasting in our daily lives. This does not mean we have to fast every day, but fasting is on our mind and a part of our lives. By spending a little time out of the day to be mindful and contemplate our relationship with IF, we further our confidence and can develop a firm grasp of our goals and aspirations. Not only is maintaining awareness of our body and mind important to our goals in this book, but also an important practice to implement every day. Our mindset and perception of a situation affect us subtly.

We emphasize awareness and mindfulness so much in this book for a good reason. We see the ancient cultures using fasting to great success, and it is certain that their practices in mindfulness and awareness are key to this success. Old practices like meditation and deep thought were very important to overall wellbeing in ancient philosophy. And so, as we see our ancestors and their practices permeating our current world, being studied in scientific settings and utilized in everyday life, we must give credit where credit is due and acknowledge that these practices are a very important aspect of existence. While keeping this in mind, let's move forward. Here, we begin the physical journey. We need to choose what type of fast works for us, schedule our meals, and then begin.

First things first, how do you want to fast? Choosing a practice type will be tough, at first, and more often than not, the first course of action is not the one we stick with. Depending on work, family, and other important influences, we can choose one of the styles in the previous chapter and work with it and see it change as we do. You can do a little customization there, some slight changes here. It is your practice, so do what you feel is best for you and not what everyone else is doing. We cannot tell you everything to do, but here are some helpful tips for the weeks leading up to the first fast:

1. **Think about it.** Think of yourself and what you want to accomplish. Consider your consumption and how it affects your body and mind. Prepare mentally for challenges that you will face – hunger, physical changes, emotions, and other drastic changes – that accompany this practice.

2. **Prepare physically.** If you find that you're are in poor health, you may want to start changing little things in the week or two leading up to the fast. Cut back on desserts and detrimental foods, take a walk and other casual exercises, or chat with friends and family about what you're trying to accomplish to find support.

3. **Meal prep.** Many people find that organizing meals beforehand helps keep them on track. Buying reusable containers and preparing a week's worth of meals to keep in the fridge helps save time and ensures you keep your diet right for the fast.

4. **Ease in.** Many feel that jumping right into a fast is shocking to their bodies, so the week before your major fast, maybe do half of what you planned for the big week. Maybe pick a fasting technique and use it for one or two days.

By preparing yourself beforehand, there's less of a chance that you will fail or have to restart the fast. You will be ready for any changes or unexpected outcomes that may find their way to you. Do not be disheartened if you cannot complete a fast the first time around. Everyone is different, and some people take the calorie restriction easier than others. If you have issues getting started, do not give up. Change your plan as you see fit, even if you only make it twenty-five percent of the week, you still have begun your transformation; you have still started changing your life for the better. The subtlest of changes have begun as soon as you started thinking about changing yourself. Be confident in yourself and your convictions. It's quite all right to fail; this is where we learn the most about ourselves. In fact, failing can even be viewed as an exercise in mindfulness. You learn from your mistakes and can try a different approach the next time around. All in all, do not give up. If you truly value yourself and your life, then this should be plenty of motivation to continue onward until you have reached your goals. Having prepared yourself mentally and physically, success is inevitable.

Once we have given our schedule, lifestyle, and personal needs some thorough thought, we need to think even deeper about our personal goals. Are you seeking simply to lose a few pounds? Are you only curious about IF and not sure about the beginning? How will starting a fasting routine affect your lifestyle and the people around you? The questions are infinite in this context, but for all our intents and purposes with this book, we have a loose set of goals that we aim to achieve:

- Ridding ourselves of excess fat
- Developing a mindful and aware perception of health
- Adjusting our diets to suit a healthful lifestyle
- Maintaining any progress we achieve (keep weight off, maintain awareness)
- Through the combination of the goals above transform our lives for the better

This list is presented as a general and vague overview of our intentions with this book. Even if you really only want to lose a few pounds, doing so will also transform your mindset and awareness, whether it's intentional or not. Develop a personal list with the above goals in mind. The list can be anything you want to change: weight loss, health, new job, new home, etc. Anything you desire, add it to this list and think about how a healthier lifestyle can affect these things. From the mundane to the most important, feel free to be as specific as you need to be with your goals. You can apply these lifestyle changes to other aspects of your life too. Improving your health is inevitably going to touch all corners of your life, so setting goals outside the scope of physical health is quite all right. As we move forward let's also take time to visualize ourselves as the people we wish to be. Visualize yourself at peak performance, visualize your life and surroundings as you truly want to be. This image will act as motivation and also as a primer for your mindfulness practice. The body and mind work together as one, so treat them as equals as we embark on our newfound Intermittent Fasting lifestyle.

Now that we have a solid idea of what we aim to achieve, we can begin taking action to start our IF routine. The guide below will take all the methods we've explored and lay out weeklong step-by-step instructions for each method.

Chapter 8: One Week Step-by-Step Guide

Now that we've gotten started and prepared our minds and bodies let's take a look at a step-by-step guide covering seven days of Intermittent Fasting. Here, we will provide a seven-day guide for each of the methods mentioned in the previous chapter. We will start the guides out with a 'preparation day', being the day before the first day of your fasting week. This day allows us to ground ourselves and prepare physically and mentally for the week to come. This guide can act as a quick reference guide during your journey, as well as a strict guideline for the various types of Intermittent Fasting.

Accompanying these guides will be some suggestions for customizing your practice. Customization techniques also come in handy to personalize your routine. A thoughtful approach to this would be to make your practice distinct and in tune with your wishes and goals. We will explore some customization techniques below, but feel free to be creative and use your best judgment. Do your research, listen to your body, and, as always, be mindful.

With the following guide, we will suggest good times for exercise according to the information we have learned over the course of this book. Let's keep in mind that this is simply a guide and does not particularly have to be followed strictly. Any suggestions for meal timing, non-caloric drinks, or exercise are only loose guidelines based on the science and studies we have analyzed. Being aware that not everyone has the same schedule, we will do our best to make the guide concise and easy to fit into your daily routine. Be creative with customization and always have plenty of water available!

The following lists will give seven-day examples for a few of the Intermittent Fasting methods mentioned above.

The 16/8 Method

Guideline:

- Fast sixteen hours per day
- Eating window eight hours per day
- Non-caloric drinks acceptable
- Stay hydrated
- Exercise first thing in the morning

With the 16/8 method, you will be fasting for around sixteen hours out of the 24-hour day, which leaves an eating window of around eight hours. Obviously, your fasting hours will include the amount of time that you sleep. We will focus on one popular arrangement of this method where your eight-hour eating window is in the evening. This is probably the easiest way to go about this method, especially if combined with exercise in the morning.

Sunday

For our guide here, you will start with Sunday. Although you are not fasting on this day, you still want to prepare yourself for the upcoming week. Be sure to remember what time your last meal is today. Sixteen hours from that time, you will begin your eating window. Have your schedule for tomorrow mentally prepared or written down. Although exercise isn't mandatory, we have discussed the added benefits of physical activity, and, for our main goal of weight loss, we will include exercise for this guide. We also would like to suggest eating light, easily digestible foods on this day for this will help you better adapt to the upcoming week. For our purposes here, let's say you finished your last meal at seven PM. This gives you until eleven AM at the earliest to have a bite to eat. You can see how this arrangement is very fitting for standard nine-to-five jobs.

Key Points:

- Remember or take note of the time of your last meal.
- Eat light, easily digestible foods on this day.
- Keep notes on the progress.

Monday (Day 1)

Morning. Upon waking up, start your day with a glass or two of water to your liking. If coffee or tea is an important part of your morning, it is fine to have as long as there is no sugar or milk added. The morning is a perfect time to exercise, the stomach is empty, and the remaining quick energy sources from any previous meals will be easily burned off, and we can start burning fat reserves. Most people will likely have to work during the week, so be sure to have access to plenty of water. We will note here that if your work requires a large amount of energy and power, this method may not be the most suitable.

Midday. If this is your first fast, you will surely be feeling the effects. Those circadian rhythms we were discussing are realizing that this is not a normal day and will adapt accordingly. Although you may feel strange, keep in mind that this is a transformative experience and will not go without some strange or unknown feelings. Noon is coming around, so we're well into our eating window. We officially have until seven PM to eat a few meals. So, have a standard lunch you would typically consume or even upgrade to a more fast-friendly meal with the suggestions for foods above. Notice the taste of your meal and really engage with the food on an intimate level. Does it feel different as you eat? Are flavors more or less intense? Keep note of any changes in perception or feeling.

After lunch, feel free to snack as you please – it's your eating window!

Evening. As the evening approaches, you can continue to snack or have meals, but most people feel comfortable having two to three meals during this time; you can adjust this to your liking. Once seven PM comes around, be sure to wind down and cease to intake any calories for the next sixteen hours.

Key Points:

- Be mindful of your body and the start of your new routine.
- Keep mental or physical notes on your experiences and changes in general.
- Stay hydrated.
- Remember the times of last caloric intake.

Tuesday (Day 2)

Morning. Upon awakening, you may repeat the previous day's routine – non-caloric drinks, exercise – but no eating until eleven AM. This morning will be very similar to Monday as we are just now starting to get into the fast. Today may be less intense as far as your body goes as it is adjusting naturally to the new IF routine. Keep notes on your morning experiences. Is it easier or more difficult to get out of bed in the morning? Are you more energetic or do you feel drained? If you have an exercise routine, is it easier or more difficult? How do you feel after the workout? Being aware of the changes you feel is important during the fasting experience. Any negative feelings or discomfort should be noted as well as positive experiences.

Midday. Your eating window approaches just in time for the standard lunchtime. As with the previous day, keep an open mind and be aware of your experiences. Again, stick with meals that you would typically eat or upgrade your meals to more nutrient-rich foods.

Evening. The second evening is here, and you're still within your eating window. Be aware of the many changes and be sure to keep up with the current pattern and be relatively strict with the routine you have.

Key Points:

- Be mindful and take notes on your feelings.
- Keep up with your routine and time patterns.
- Stay hydrated.

Wednesday (Day 3)

Morning. The third morning commences, and the routine is becoming a part of your normal routine. With all the intense writing online about the dangers of IF, we approach the third morning noticing that this transformative practice is really not that difficult but simply requires a little attention to detail and self-discipline. Live the morning as you do, go about the day as usual, and pay attention to any changes or feelings that are notable.

Midday. Lunchtime approaches once again, and we stick with our routine. Keep the meals balanced and have your snacks handy for the eight-hour window.

Evening. The third evening will be similar to the second and subsequent evenings. You have your dinner and desired snacks, but nothing past seven PM except water.

Key Points:

- Be mindful and take notes.
- Stay with your determined eating patterns.
- Stay hydrated.

Thursday (Day 4)

Morning. Similar to previous days, be mindful of your awakening and take note of any feelings, positive or negative. Keep hydrated and be appreciative and excited for your eating window.

Midday. The beginning of the eating window on this day is a milestone. You are halfway through the first week, and the practice is becoming comfortable and not unlike any other routine before you discovered fasting. Have your standard lunch and snacks. Be mindful and smile!

Evening. Trekking on through the halfway point, this night is much like the previous ones – a nice dinner and halt your caloric intake at seven PM. This evening is a good one to note any differences in your sleeping patterns. Are you falling asleep more easily? Are you sleeping through the night?

Key Points:

- Stay mindful and take notes.
- Contemplate the halfway mark.
- Stay within your eating patterns.
- Stay hydrated.

Friday (Day 5)

Morning. TGIF and another beautiful morning as usual. Be mindful and aware, stay hydrated, and continue with your day until eleven AM when you get to enjoy some food.

Midday. Eleven AM rolls around, and it's time for a snack or meal. Enjoy and take notes of any excitement you feel about your first weekend of fasting. Eat as you wish and stay hydrated.

Evening. The evening approaches and many people are taking advantage of the weekend – going out for drinks and music, etc. You have your allotted time for eating, so if you enjoy an alcoholic drink sometimes, feel free to have one but not after seven PM. (Of course, if you feel comfortable, you can intake calories past seven PM, but be sure to keep track of the time you intake your last calories and adjust the time for Saturday accordingly.)

Key Points:

- Stay mindful and take notes.

- Stay within eating patterns.
- Consider alcohol and social life and how it can affect the patterns.
- Stay hydrated. (optional)

Saturday (Day 6)

Morning. Your first weekend morning with the new fast and all is well. You may have the day off today and find yourself trying to fill the time since you are not preparing and planning as much food as usual. This morning is a great time to think about adding an exercise routine or explore other changes you may want to make for next week.

Midday. A free day is a great time to have a hike or run errands to fill time. Take note of whether or not the fasting has affected minuscule tasks like grocery shopping. Do the foods at the store seem more or less appealing? Are you less stressed while running errands or spending time in the car? A day off is a great time to really analyze the subtle transformation that is taking place. Keep your routine and only intake calories during a predetermined time slot.

Evening. The day off is coming to a close, and you have some dinner and perhaps a drink to ease into the night. This evening will seem especially exciting as you enter into Sunday and start your second week.

Key Points:

- Be aware and mindful, and don't forget to take notes.
- Consider days off and the extra free time you have.
- Stay hydrated.

Sunday (Day 7)

Whether your eighth day falls on a Sunday or not, this day is good to reflect on the past week. Look over any notes you've taken mentally or physically and see if you want to make any changes for the upcoming week. Keep your eating schedule during this time as well, although fun customization for this day could be what is known as a 'cheat' day, where you ignore you fasting practice and eat whenever you like. Another form of a cheat day would be simply to eliminate the exercise portion of the day. For our purposes of weight loss and transformation, we will stick with our routine and practice, so the eating window remains from eleven AM to seven PM.

You have completed your first official week of IF using the 16/8 method! For the following weeks, you can continue to keep up this pattern or even customize or switch to a different method. Always remember: this is your practice to improve your life. Make it your own and continue to keep notes on your progress and feelings. Don't be afraid to feel proud and accomplished with your new routine. Share the joys with coworkers and friends, and most importantly, enjoy the new and ever-changing you!

The 5/2 Method

As we discussed earlier, this method looks more like a diet than a fast, but instead of restricting certain foods, you are restricting the time frame in which you enjoy these foods. The 5/2 method involves having meals as you typically would but choosing two days of the week to consume less than 600 calories for the entire day. For this seven-day guideline, we will approach it as a standard work week, with Saturdays and Sundays as the days off.

Sunday

We start our guide on Sunday to take time to prepare for the upcoming week. Today, you should make sure you are stocked up on groceries and have the next seven days loosely scheduled. Prepping the meals for the calorie-restricted days is an excellent way to control caloric intake. Some questions of whether or not you need to make dietary changes or add some physical activity to your normal routine: *Is my typical diet nutrient-rich? Do I stay hydrated throughout the day? How much exercise do I get each week?* These questions will help alter and optimize your fasting experience. You also need to choose which two days of the week you are going to restrict caloric intake. These two days can be together like Tuesday-Wednesday or a day or two apart, such as Tuesday and Thursday, which will be the days we choose for this guide. Exercise for this guide, in particular, will be performed in the morning. Take time today to be mindful of the upcoming week and take notes of your feelings and experiences going into this new routine.

Monday (Day 1)

You awake to your first week on the 5/2 method to business as usual. Treat this day like any other; you can eat how you typically do, exercise as you normally do, and go about your day. If you feel that you have an unhealthy diet, then switching to some more nutrient dense foods will only help this process. And likewise, if you do not typically exercise, then adding some light stretching or a short walk in the morning is a good idea. If you feel that you do not ingest enough water, now is a great time to start being stricter on hydration; otherwise, this would be just a normal Monday. Be aware and mindful of how you are feeling today and take note of any new experiences the changes you make to your routine may bring.

Once the evening comes, prepare your mind and body for your first calorie-restricted day tomorrow, also your 600 calories for that day. Whether you're choosing two small meals or to snack throughout the day, have them prepared so that you will not need to worry about it tomorrow. For this guide, we will be choosing two small meals. Also, keep in mind that the transition from a typical day to restricted day will be easier the more similar the diets are day to day. For example, eating 4,000 calories today then only 600 tomorrow will be a much tougher transition than a calorie count that is closer to an average amount, around 2,000 calories.

Tuesday (Day 2)

You awake on your first calorie-restricted day. Take note on how your mindset will be: are you confident in your ability to succeed? Are you excited for this new journey? Taking notes to compare to future mornings is highly recommended. So, you start your day by drinking plenty of water, some light exercise of your choosing, and you will opt out of breakfast today.

Once lunchtime approaches, you can enjoy one of your small 300-calorie meals or snacks. Be aware of how enjoyable such a small meal can be: are you excited about this meal even knowing it's small and there's not much more to come? Is the small amount discouraging? Although it's not as much as you're used to, your body knows something is new and will adapt. Have plenty of water if you do not feel full and continue with the day.

The evening approaches, and it's time for another meal. Are you excited for this meal? Do you feel hungry? Analyze this first dinner and be truthful with yourself. You may desire more food but be strong and fill up on water or perhaps some non-caffeinated tea or coffee. Take note of similar experiences for bedtime: are you falling asleep easier? Are you thinking about more food? Be reassured that tomorrow is a normal day and you can eat what you like.

Wednesday (Day 3)

Another normal day as you arise. Before you hit the kitchen for breakfast, take note of how you feel and perhaps contemplate it over your light morning exercise. Now, you can have a meal as per usual and go about your day, periodically stopping and taking the time to be mindful and aware of any new experiences.

This day will continue like a typical day. In the evening, be sure to have your 600 calories planned out for tomorrow, and again, be aware of your bedtime experiences.

Thursday (Day 4)

Your second morning of calorie-restricted intake is a milestone. You have made it halfway through the first week of your new life. This day will be identical to Tuesday (Day 2) as you will be having two 300-calorie meals. Of course, if you wish to change the time of the day, you have your meals, and that's fine. For this guide, we will stick with exercise this morning with plenty of water and an optional non-caloric drink (coffee, tea) but no meal until lunch.

Lunchtime approaches and you're ready for the meal. Enjoy it and be aware of how this new routine makes you feel. Be mindful of the flavors and ask yourself similar questions just like Tuesday.

The evening approaches and you see your second meal in the near future. Be aware of your feelings leading up to the meal and continue being aware of any new experiences. Treat bedtime the same with mindfulness and awareness.

Friday (Day 5)

Today, you awake and treat it like the previous mornings – exercise, hydration, and mindfulness. However, you get to eat normally, so enjoy breakfast and lunch accordingly.

Once the evening comes, you are aware that weekends are spent relaxing, maybe with alcoholic drinks and socializing. This is permitted since today is not a restricted day.

Saturday (Day 6)

This day is similar to yesterday. Although it is a day off and you have no restrictions on caloric intake, continue being mindful of your new routine: *Do I want to change or intensify next week's practice? Do I feel comfortable with the new routine?* Spend this day off as you normally would but with your new lifestyle in the back of your mind.

Sunday (Day 7)

This is the final day of the seven-day week. Treat this day as you would any – no calorie restriction or boundaries, just a basic day off before the work week begins again. Did you decide to alter the routine from last week? If so, make sure you have meals prepared and have the schedule all worked out for your upcoming second week with the 5/2 method.

Upon completion of the first week, what subtle changes have you seen in yourself and body? Do you feel that this week was a success? Take a deep breath and congratulate yourself on a new journey, and make a commitment to stay on a mindful path for the foreseeable future.

The Eat Stop Eat Method

This method of IF is a little more taxing on the body as it requires a full 24-hour fast one or two times a week. The fast itself asks you not to consume any calories for a full 24 hours. So, essentially, the only thing you will ingest is water. Non-caloric drinks are acceptable as well, such as coffee and tea. The non-caloric drinks should not have milk or sugar added to them and also be aware of caffeine content in these drinks, especially with an empty stomach. And since this method is slightly more intensive, you need to be even more cautious as a beginner approaching this style of fasting.

Sunday

While preparing for the 'eat stop eat' method, you need to take a serious look at your previous relationship with fasting and food itself. If you have no previous experience with calorie restriction, it is recommended that you experiment with it, perhaps with one of the other methods in this book, to make sure you are comfortable with a full day of no calorie intake. It is also important that when you are having meals during the next seven days that you eat food that your body is used to having. Eat your usual diet and similar foods. With this caution on your mind, you can proceed to prepare your upcoming week.

So today, your responsibilities include preparing your mind and body for the upcoming week of IF. Going without calories for 24 hours is something your body has generally not experienced your whole life, but be reminded that it can be safely practiced and has been safely practiced for centuries. First of all, you need to decide the day(s) that you are choosing to fast on. For this guide, we will be fasting for two days out of the week, Tuesday (Day 2) and Thursday (Day 4). These days, of course, can be changed at your convenience and preference. Once you have selected your days, contemplate and plan your days.

While considering your next week, you need to take into consideration your diet. If you have a poor diet, then it may be a good idea to change your diet to the guidelines in the previous chapter for a week or two before the IF begins. Although you are fasting on only two days, the week itself should still be viewed as a part of the fasting practice. You need to make sure you have your proper groceries and plenty of water. To optimize the week, you can even meal prep and prepare your meals for each day and have them ready to go in the refrigerator or other storage. Remain mindful and listen to your body. As you spend this day like any other, you will keep the beginning of your transformational week in mind well into the evening and off to bed.

Monday (Day 1)

Luckily, for one of the more intensive fasts in this book, the eat stop eat method requires you to eat precisely what you would normally eat on non-fast days. This fast asks that you do not dramatically alter your normal eating schedule on the non-fast days as to avoid putting too much strain and change on your body in such a short amount of time. This will make the non-fasting days pretty simple, but you also need to maintain your awareness and mindfulness throughout the week even on days when you can eat. And so, for Monday, simply go about your day as usual while ensuring your mind is prepared for the calorie-restricted day tomorrow. It is recommended to eat on the lighter side of your normal diet tonight and, of course, keep very hydrated.

Tuesday (Day 2)

You awake on your first full fast day mentally prepared and ready to take on this new practice. Taking plenty of water first thing in the morning and accompanying some light exercise is ideal. If you must have caffeine in the morning, the acceptable drinks are coffee and tea as long as it is not sweetened or mixed with other additives. Regardless of how you spend your day, you need to be sure that you have access to plenty of water throughout the day. Consistently drink water, but don't consume it too quickly.

This is the plan for the entire day. No calories, just water. As simple as it is, you may be craving food as your body is used to meals at certain times. This may be uncomfortable, at first, but stay busy and keep in mind that you are trying to reset your body's rhythms. One aspect of the completely restricted day is all the free time you have. If you're working on this day, it may not be as noticeable. However, once you arrive home, there will be plenty of free time. Try to stay busy by having planned activities to do; a casual walk, household chores, games, and media come in handy with the extra time not spent preparing and cooking meals.

As evening falls and you prepare for sleep, look back on your first fast day and analyze your experiences: did the lack of food aggravate you? How do you feel physically? Do things seem altered in some way? These questions help to keep track of your experiences and recall them for comparison later after your second fast day. If you have trouble falling asleep, a book or light stretching helps greatly.

Wednesday (Day 3)

The third day of your IF week will be very similar to the first. But when you first awake, be conscious of how you feel with such an empty stomach: is it difficult or easier to get out of bed? Do you feel lighter? Are you terribly eager to have some food? Start the day with light exercise and water and eat as you normally would – having a similar calorie intake as the first day of this week. Take note of how the food tastes and how it feels entering your body after a day of no eating. This day will continue as normal with mindfulness and awareness of your next fast day.

Thursday (Day 4)

Your second and final fully restricted day of the week is upon you. Much like Day 2, you will begin with plenty of water and light exercise in the morning, optional caffeinated non-caloric drinks, and mindfulness. Again, consistently take note of your experiences and feelings. This day shouldn't be any more difficult than the first calorie-restricted day – since you have a general idea of what to expect. As such, you will have access to plenty of water and keep hydrated throughout the day, paying attention to your experiences and staying busy.

As the evening approaches, you will spend the time keeping your mind occupied and preparing for a full night's sleep.

Friday (Day 5)

This day will begin similar to Day 3 in that you will take note of how you feel in the morning and how waking with an empty stomach affects you physically and mentally. You have completed your calorie-restricted days for the week, but keep your experiences fresh on your mind and contemplate them over the weekend. Today and the next, you will be on your regular eating schedule as well.

Saturday (Day 6)

This day will be identical to yesterday, and you will remain on your normal eating schedule. Today, you will also decide if you want to keep your same IF regimen for next week. Taking into consideration all your experiences from the past six days, you need to ask yourself: *was this week a success? Will I keep this Intermittent Fasting method for the upcoming week or try a different approach? Did the days I chose to fast fit my schedule conveniently?* Once you have answered these questions, you can go about your day as usual.

Sunday (Day 7)

Now, you have hit Day 7, and you should have a general idea of what you want to do as far as fasting is concerned for the next seven days. You will prepare for the upcoming week accordingly and ensure you have the proper supplies and schedule.

Added Notes on the Eat Stop Eat Method

Having explored this method of IF thoroughly, you can alter this method in many ways. One way to step up the intensity of the practice is to push the calorie-restricted days together and go an entire 48 hours without the caloric intake. Not only is this a great way to ensure the body uses reserved fat energy, but it is also a great test of the mind and your commitment to your transformation. The two days together is not recommended for beginners and will require much thought and dedication to yourself and this respected practice.

Alternate Day Method

The alternate day method requires that you alternate your fast days every other day – that is if you didn't restrict calories today, then tomorrow you are to restrict calories in some manner. This method is great to customize for your practice. For our guide here, we will be borrowing from the 5/2 diet and cut back your calorie intake to less than 600 calories on fasting days. You will approach this method in the guide as a standard work week with Saturday and Sundays being days off, but, of course, synchronize this practice up with your schedule accordingly. In this guide, your first restricted day will be Tuesday.

Sunday

As with the previous guides, you will begin with the day before your first official day to contemplate and prepare for the upcoming week. You need to make sure you have plenty of groceries and access to water and that you are mentally prepared for the practice you're about to commit to. Prepping meals works great for this method as you can prepare a meal with the desired number of calories beforehand and have them ready to go in the refrigerator. This helps to control your calorie intake and allows you not to have to worry about preparing food throughout the week as you navigate the IF terrain. As you prepare for this week, be mindful and aware of what you are committing to and get plenty of rest tonight.

Monday (Day 1)

Today will be like any normal day. You will wake up and have your standard morning routine. If exercise isn't a part of this routine, this week is a good time to add it in. Plenty of water as needed and you will go about your day, and as usual, keeping in mind that tomorrow is a restricted intake day. If you are changing your diet as well this week, this method asks that you do not dramatically alter your non-fast days too wildly, but adding nutrient-rich foods is always a good idea regardless of what week it is. Having another normal day complete, you spend the evening mentally preparing for tomorrow, keeping note of your experiences and anticipation.

Tuesday (Day 2)

Morning. Your first restricted intake day begins as you awake. Plenty of water and light exercise is on the agenda for the morning. Coffee and tea are acceptable, but be aware of any calories you're adding with sugars and milk as you are only ingesting around 600 calories today in a two-meal approach. Contemplate your experience this morning: *am I excited about my new practice? Do I feel that my new routine is in sync with the rest of my life?* You complete your morning and move along to lunchtime.

Midday. As midday approaches, you can have your first 300-calorie meal for the day. As you begin the meal, analyze your experience: *is this a satisfying amount of food? Did I make proper choices for the contents of this meal? How does this experience differ from other lunches in my recent past?* You complete lunch and continue with your day as usual, being aware of how your body feels and staying hydrated.

Evening. Once nightfall approaches, you can enjoy your dinner, another 300-calorie meal comprised of nutrient-dense foods loosely based on the guidelines in Chapter 6. With this meal, you near the end of your first calorie-restricted day. Think about your experience: *what were the hours in between meals like? Am I still craving food after this evening meal? How enjoyable was the food with such restricted intake*? With bedtime approaching, focus on your mind and body, keeping note of any feelings or experiences as you fall asleep.

Wednesday (Day 3)

This morning will be like Day 1, although you are waking up to a calorie-restricted body. You will have plenty of water and light exercise, then continue your day with a normal intake of food and drink while keeping consistent attention to any new experiences and feelings. You stay aware that tomorrow is a restricted intake day and you should consider yesterday: *were the meals up to par? Could I slightly alter tomorrow to optimize my practice?* Feel free to customize as you wish; this is your IF practice.

Thursday (Day 4)

This day will be identical to Day 2 unless you decide to make any changes. For this guide, we will keep to your set guidelines and treat this day the same as Day 2 – water and light exercise in the morning, a 300-calorie meal for lunch, and a 300-calorie meal for dinner. All the while taking note of your experiences and being mindful of your changes.

Friday (Day 5)

Similar to Days 1 and 3, Day 5 is a day to go about your normal eating schedule. Spend the day on your regular schedule and eat meals similar to Days 1 and 3. As you continue to alternate days, be aware of how the practice differs on calorie-restricted days: *how was Day 1 different from Day 5? Has calorie restriction become easier to practice? How are my energy levels?* By comparing the days and actively engaging with the experiences, you can get a firm grip on how you want your IF practice to evolve.

Saturday (Day 6)

As a day that is not a calorie-restricted day, you will go about your business as usual, eating meals similar to Days 2 and 4, maintaining awareness of your IF even on this non-fast day. As you can see, the alternating day method allows you to maintain a nice pattern that is easy to keep track of. This method is noticeably great for beginners with its easy to follow guidelines and excellent flexibility. Treat this day as a celebratory one as well as you near the end of your first week of IF. Perhaps treat yourself to a sweet treat or a night out with friends.

Sunday (Day 7)

Today is a calorie-restricted day to be treated like Days 1, 3, and 5. The morning is spent drinking water and some light exercise.

Lunch is a 300-calorie nutrient-rich meal, and dinner is also a 300-calorie nutrient-rich meal.

You must also decide if you are going to continue this pattern for the upcoming week. If you find that this practice is working, then you will continue alternating days for the next week or even month! Keeping this pattern solid for many weeks will inevitably lead to this diet being your normal practice and seem like any other day compared to the days that filled this past week. Customize as you wish and, of course, always stay mindful and aware of what your body is telling you.

Warrior Method

Our next method is the warrior method. Named in regards to Paleo diets and warrior tribes of ancient man, this method calls for meals that are as raw and unprocessed as possible. If your diet is not in line with this guideline, it may help to adhere to a Paleo-like diet the week before beginning this method.

The warrior method is a relatively simple one to follow as it does not require any days that are one hundred percent calorie-restricted. This method of IF involves one huge meal in the evening time while simply eating raw and unprocessed snacks throughout the day or just no calories throughout the day. For our guide in this book, you will casually snack during the day and have a big nutrient-rich meal in the evening. You will treat the upcoming week as a typical work week with a standard weekend.

Sunday

The day before you begin your warrior fast, you need to spend the day preparing your body and mind for the changes and new routine you are approaching this week. Ensure that you have plenty of unprocessed snack foods readily available; nuts, fruits, and veggies are ideal for the daytime snacking. Access to plenty of water and a general idea of what you wish to have for large evening meals is a must. As you get ready for bed, consider your ancient ancestors and their very raw, unprocessed diet. Also, maintain your mindful and confident approach to this new routine of IF.

Monday (Day 1)

Daytime. The first day of your method will be started with plenty of water and light exercise. As mentioned, you will be snacking throughout the day, so you may enjoy your raw foods as you wish. For this guide, you will be having a very light breakfast of raw foods and perhaps a tea or coffee as well. As the day rolls on, you can have tiny amounts of nuts and berries throughout, being cautious not to eat a whole day's worth of snacks in one sitting.

As lunchtime approaches, maintain this mentality – only having snacks here and there through the day. Be mindful of the experiences you face: are you craving the other snacks you've prepared? Are you having a hard time not eating all your supplies? How would tiny snacks compare to no food at all?

Nighttime. The evening approaches, and you can start considering your first big meal of the week. Preparing it should require minimal cooking, so feel free to be creative. Steaming foods instead of frying is a great way to stay in line with these guidelines. This meal can be whatever you wish but stay within the structure of the least processed foods – no frozen meals, no fast foods, and no deep frying. Avoiding as much prepackaged food as possible is key. With this in mind, there is an upside that this meal is meant to be huge. Feel free to fill your belly nice and full of nutrient-rich foods this evening. Keep a note on how your body reacts to this: do you feel full more quickly or with less food than usual? Is raw food as enjoyable as your normal choices for dinner? Note these experiences as you are going to compare each evening's experiences as you move through the week. It helps to have similar meals through this week as well, but it's not mandatory.

Tuesday (Day 2)

Daytime. The second day and all subsequent days for that matter are very similar to Day 1. This method requires consistency and a real focus on how raw your foods are, which has not been an issue for the previous methods in this book. With this in mind, you start Day 2 just like Day 1; plenty of water, light exercise, and if you so choose, a very light raw snack, preferably fruits, veggies, and nuts. On with the day, you continue to snack. Compare this day to yesterday: *do I* *feel any different? Am I adapting easily to only having raw snacks during the day?* Keep a close watch on how your day-to-day experience changes subtly as you continue the warrior method.

Nighttime. This evening will be very similar to last night. Prepare a large meal as unprocessed as possible and as nutrient-rich as possible. Although the evenings like this are going to repeat, be very aware of any changes in your experience and relationship with the larger meals: *am I excited to enjoy this meal? How have I adapted to the new raw diet?* Continue this evaluation consistently through the week every night before and after the meal.

Wednesday (Day 3)

Daytime. As mentioned earlier, this method is about consistency and maintaining an unprocessed diet. So naturally, Day 3 looks identical to the previous days; plenty of water and light exercise in the morning, snacking lightly on raw foods throughout the day, and the ever-important mindfulness and awareness as you see subtle changes in your mind and body.

Nighttime. Another similar night approaches and you anticipate another unprocessed meal. Keeping the large meal similar in caloric intake and size, you move onward on your warrior journey, keeping note of those subtle changes and experiences each day.

Thursday (Day 4)

Daytime. Day 4 is like any other during this repetitious week: water and exercise fill the morning and raw snacking all day in tiny amounts. By this time in the week, the changes may be less subtle as your body adapts into its new routine. Continue the process, confident and aware.

Nighttime. This evening is like the previous ones. If you feel a little bored of the similar meals, always remember that this is your practice and you can customize as you like. Just try your hardest not to venture too far outside of the structures and patterns that you have established.

Friday (Day 5)

Daytime. Another morning of hydration and light exercise. You've made it one work week, so how are you feeling? Are there any noticeable changes physically or mentally? Continue your snacking guidelines and keep the mindfulness at the forefront of your thoughts.

Nighttime. This evening is just like the others, but it is the weekend, so maybe reward your dedication with a night out for drinks or socializing to break up the monotony of this method. Maintain your awareness and see if there are any new changes in the way you view a social setting or a casual glass of wine at home.

Saturday (Day 6)

Daytime. Day 6 remains unchanged compared to the previous days. It is a weekend, so if you wish, you can skip exercise, but plenty of water and keep on snacking as per usual. At this point, the patterns should seem pretty set into place in your mind and body, but take this day to look back on the week: *is the warrior method working for my lifestyle? How has my mind and body changed in just one week? Is this new practice creating new paths in my day-to-day life?* Consider if you wish to continue this method for next week and take your time as you analyze the past six days.

Nighttime. Time for another large meal, again maintaining the structure and guidelines as much as possible. Once bedtime approaches, you should have a firm grasp on whether or not you are continuing this method or any other changes coming for next week.

Sunday (Day 7)

You have managed to keep your IF protocol under control for a full week now. How different do you feel compared to seven days ago? You will still treat this day as a warrior fast day but will take action in making necessary adjustments for the upcoming week. Any groceries or other suitable supplies need to be available, and you should be aware of any alterations you are making this week. Perhaps you wish to change your snacking options? Maybe you need a 'cheat' day once a week for now? All the possible customizations are endless as you analyze your needs and desires. With that in mind, you approach another large meal and can start implementing your changes as soon as you wish or simply keep going with your established patterns for as many weeks as you like.

Spontaneity Method

We now move on to our final example of IF methods. The spontaneity method is pretty self-explanatory: you may spontaneously choose when to fast as you see fit. Not feeling hungry today? Restrict calories. Feel like only eating raw foods today? Make it happen. Simply want to cut out sweets for a week? Easy. The endless possibilities with this method make it great for beginners who wish to experiment with different methods to see what feels right. It also works for busy people and parents who want to keep a mindful approach to health but don't have the schedule to adhere to strict guidelines and rules. And sure, this may seem like you're only skipping meals because it's convenient or a lazy way to fast, but if we can funnel our perception of our diets and lifestyles through an 'intermittent fasting lens' by maintaining mindfulness and awareness about our bodies and how fasting affects them, then we will find that a spontaneous method can work just as well as any other. To reiterate, no one way works for everyone, and some people thrive under less structured conditions.

For this method, you will not require a day-by-day guide since that would contradict the purpose of spontaneity. You will, however, explore some ideas and suggestions for this method.

Being spontaneous can have an amazing effect on the mind. It adds a sense of freedom to a monotonous week or month and can really help people relax and live in the moment. When it comes to fasting, it works the same way. Go with your gut; if you feel strongly about just eating some delicious fruit all day, do it and call it a part of your fasting routine. Often, when this practice is put into play seriously, use a pattern, and structure forms in itself, and the practitioner finds themselves having a solid IF routine without even trying to. While also taking ideas from the previously mentioned methods, here are some ideas to throw into your spontaneous practice:

- Go with your gut; if you feel it, do it.
- 24-hour calorie restriction. Waking up feeling like a day fast? Make it happen.
- Not hungry when you wake up? Skip breakfast and/or lunch.
- Feel like you've had too much sugar lately? Cut out sweets or alcohol for a set duration of time.
- Blink and the day has flown by without food? Call it a fast and go to bed.
- Does your religion or spiritual preference have a holiday that traditionally requires fasting? Try it out.

The list could go forever, but keep in mind the serious nature of fasting and always approach it with your overall wellbeing in mind. You can take this method and make your own rules but always accompany these rules with research and contemplation. Also, it is good to state that although this method is a free form, it is not particularly a good idea to use the easy-going nature of this fast as an excuse not to stay with your convictions. If you state to yourself that you are fasting or planning to, stick with it. Commitment and dedication are two of the most important factors and lessons of IF.

We have officially explored some of the more popular methods of Intermittent Fasting. These guidelines will act as a great stepping stone to your customized methods if you decide to stay with the IF lifestyle. As you continue on this journey, always maintain mindfulness and awareness about your body and mind.

Chapter 9: Dos and Don'ts of Intermittent Fasting

All the myths and broad array of opinions about the subject can make fasting research a nightmare on the Internet, but don't be disheartened by people online and stay focused on your goals. This doesn't mean to go headfirst into it without being aware of the dangers that can come with a haphazard practice. Keeping a keen eye out for red flags from your body is important. Safety is overall the most important thing when it comes to these transformative practices and, of course, we're trying to improve our health not destroy it.

The following list will serve as a quick reference guide to safe Intermittent Fasting. If you have any doubts or questions that remain unanswered in this book, the following guide should give insight and act as a general basis for the unwritten rules of fasting. With all the information we have explored throughout this book, you should be readily prepared to begin an IF regimen, but, as with anything in life, there can be unexpected twists and turns. If there are any doubts in your mind, expand your research or consult your physician for advice. And, as always, your body knows best; do what feels right but also consider this list.

Do make sure you are fit to fast. There are plenty of physical conditions that should not be combined with IF. You should not be fasting if:

- You are pregnant or lactating.
- You have diabetes.
- You are under the age of eighteen.
- You have a serious medical condition.
- You are taking prescription drugs that may have unpredictable results while fasting.

Do let your friends and family know you are fasting. Not only is spending time with friends and family a great way to spend downtime during a fast but having their support will also help you attain your goals. Be sure to let them know all about fasting if they are not familiar with the practice. This can help the uninformed understand the practice so that they don't think you're starving yourself. Also, in some cases, your friends and family may be interested in starting an IF practice themselves and having a fasting partner just makes it a little easier.

Do let your primary care provider know that you are interested in fasting. He or she will need to know this to customize their approach to treating you. The transformative nature of IF should be handled with great care, and your doctor, knowing this information, will be key to optimizing the effects of the fast.

Do take vitamins as needed. Depending on the method of fasting you choose, you may feel the need to supplement your vitamins and minerals. Since you're cutting back on the amount of food you're consuming, you may need a little extra help replacing some nutrients you would normally rely on. It is not mandatory to supplement; it's not for everyone, but it is safe to do so. Most certainly consult your physician if you have other questions about the supplements.

Do prepare your mind and body. We stress this a lot throughout the book, but it is a very important point that needs to be addressed. By asking yourself tough questions like, "Am I ready to dedicate myself to this fast?" will allow you to see what needs to be done to prepare yourself for the fast. Actively thinking about your intentions and goals goes a long way to analyze your lifestyle and what you want to get out of an IF practice. Meditation, yoga, and improving your diet during the weeks leading up to the fast are only going to help you ease into the transformation.

Do prepare your home. If your home is full of junk food and other tempting things that could jeopardize your success, it is recommended that you rid yourself of these things. This is not only a practice in maintaining self-control but of also cleansing your house of your past. This is a part of the transformation process and does wonders to make your home feel spacious and uncluttered. Maybe rearrange your furniture the way you intend to rearrange your health. Hang positive and welcoming décor, and overall, let your surrounding change with you.

Do plan your fasting days. You want to make sure that the week(s) you choose to fast are ones that will be relatively stress-free and not the busiest week/s of the year. Planning a fast during a holiday that involves sweets and feasts is setting yourself up for failure. Planning a fast during a marathon you intend to run is just asking for trouble. Ensure there are no major events that will hinder your focus on attaining your goals with IF.

Do have fun. Be proud that you're taking control of your health with IF. You will come across skeptics and critics, but stay focused on what you need. This is your practice; it is a part of you, and it aims to improve your overall quality of life. Be confident. Be happy. Be yourself.

Don't forget about water. It's no secret how important water is to everyday living, but during a fast, it is even more important. Staying hydrated should be at the forefront of your mind through the entire fast. This mentality should carry over into everyday life. Drink water. Easy.

Don't stress out. You've probably heard of the slang term 'hangry'. It's used to describe being angry because you're hungry. Although not the most scientific of terms, going without our normal food intake can sometimes lead to stress. Through the stress, many undesired and misunderstood emotions can come through leading to a vicious cycle. When you feel stressed, take five to ten deep breaths or, if possible, walk it off around the block. Your body will get used to the calorie restriction, and these sudden stressors will subside.

Don't overindulge the night before a fast. Depending on the fasting method, it is safe to say that stuffing yourself full of food the night before a fast is counterintuitive. Stuffing your stomach contradicts the entire goal of this practice – developing awareness about your body and shedding excess fat. Try to balance out your mindset a bit by preparing your body for the fast by eating light the night before.

Don't celebrate the end of your fast by overindulging. You may feel starved after a fasting week, but that's no reason to go out drinking heavily or indulging in fried foods. Sure, a treat here and there won't hurt, but don't use your fasting practice as an excuse to be unhealthy. This attitude will build a toxic relationship with your fasting routine. If you want to get a little crazy, do so because you're a little crazy, not because you finished a fast. This potentially can send you right back to where you began.

Don't be afraid to stop your fast. If you find yourself feeling ill or other discomforts during a fast, cut it short. Your health is what is most important, so take any measures possible to avoid harm. It may feel like a defeat, but you can try again in the near future once the issue is resolved. There's no sense is risking great harm just because you want to finish a fast.

This list may not cover all the experiences you will encounter on your journey, but we did touch base on many common mistakes and important things that often get overlooked. Be sure always to consider all the possible outcomes when planning a fast; this is why we put so much emphasis on contemplating and analyzing our experiences while we practice intermittent fasting. Overall the most important aspect of these awareness-enhancing practices is to listen to your body. If you feel more discomfort or especially pain, don't hesitate to postpone your fast until a later date. Consulting your physician is recommended if you experience any concerning pain or discomfort.

Conclusion

Thank you for making it through to the end of *Intermittent Fasting for Women: An Essential Guide to Weight Loss, Fat-Burning, and Healing Your Body Without Sacrificing All Your Favorite Foods*. It should have been informative and provided you with all of the tools you need to achieve your goals – whatever they might be.

As we come to a close, we hope you are feeling prepared for the transformative process that is about to begin. There is much related content about this kind of fasting out in the world and surely more to come as its popularity grows, but this comprehensive book serves as an unbiased and welcoming breath of fresh air in the world of Intermittent Fasting.

A simple glance at the history of Intermittent Fasting and the incredible impact it has had on our world and culture is very evident. As far back into our past as we can see, humans have implemented fasting into their culture for a variety of reasons. Spiritual and religious endeavors use fasting rituals and practices as a means of devotion and insight into the unknown realms that humans have considered since the dawn of time. Fasting has been used as a means to ensure survival in many cultures after food harvests were depleted, leading to long-lived societies yielding residents that are living examples of longevity and health. Right up to the present day, fasting remains a staple in indigenous cultures and technologically advantageous societies alike.

As scientists continue to study the effects of Intermittent Fasting on the body and brain, they confirm the value of this amazing practice and solidify its role as a positive health practice whose benefits are seemingly endless. As we conclude this book and continue with our personal practice, we keep in mind the history, influence, and newfound scientific backing that validates Intermittent Fasting as a legitimate, beneficial health practice. The foundation that Intermittent Fasting has built for itself is one that is unshakeable as it moves swiftly into the mainstream culture of the Western world.

As you achieve your goals with these methods, the next step is to continue with your routine, changing it as your life changes, transforming with it as it is a part of you now. Keeping a journal on your experiences comes in handy too – see your progress and be proud, feel accomplished, and live to the fullest. Sharing your experience with others can also be important; sometimes, the only thing someone needs to start their journey is a personal friend to discuss and inform them of the wonders of the Intermittent Fasting lifestyle.

Part 2: Keto Diet

How to Use the Ketogenic Diet to Lose Weight, Burn Fat, and Increase Mental Clarity, Including How to Get into Ketosis and Fasting on Keto for Beginners

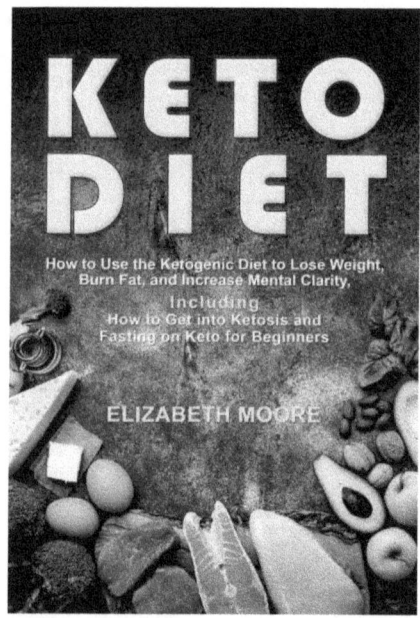

Introduction

The following chapters will discuss how you can easily and smoothly transition from your regular diet to the keto diet, a diet that is driven by eating low-carbs and high fats. It has a ton of benefits, including weight loss, more energy, better workouts, and a sharper and better focus. No matter what your reasons are for checking out the keto diet, you will find these in here and more.

This book will go over more than just the science and the idea of the keto diet. It will also go into the benefits, myths, truths, exercising on a diet, what the keto flu is and how to deal with it, and a whole bunch of other information you might need.

The idea of this book is not to list a whole bunch of recipes and tell you just to eat this; you will work this out. There is nobody here telling you what you should be eating and when you should be eating. The idea is to give you the information you need to help yourself start to find the foods you like and cook the way you want to cook. This book will help you put together a meal plan that you will love, and look forward to cooking.

Chapter 1: The Beginning

How does the keto diet work, and why is it so different from other diets?

The keto diet is when you train your body to use primarily the fats that you eat for energy. You take control of your metabolism that way, putting in motion a process called Ketosis. Ketosis uses the fats that you consume to create the energy your body needs.

That's the short explanation. Here's the long one:

In the basic sense, the keto diet is typically one of low carbs, moderate protein, and high fats. This causes the body to produce what are called ketones. Now, because you probably don't know what "ketones" means, here is a list of vocabulary you should know before you get started. It will make things easier to understand for later on.

Ketones: The chemicals that emerge and multiply once you start burning fat for energy. They are converted from stored body fat in the liver. The more you eat more fat and fewer carbs, the more your body will produce them.

Carbs: Also known as carbohydrates, carbs are molecules that contain carbon, hydrogen, and oxygen atoms. They are also one of the three macronutrients. The other two are fat and protein.

Glucose: You might be more familiar with its other name, blood sugar. Glucose is the chemical that is the easiest to break down in the body, making it an easy source of energy. Glucose gets converted into glycogen, which is stored for energy use. Excess glucose gets converted into fat stores.

Insulin: A hormone made in the pancreas. Insulin is what the body needs to break down sugar, or glucose, or carbs. Insulin is necessary for your body, as it is used to help keep your blood sugar from getting too high or too low. Diabetes is when your pancreas can no longer create insulin.

Carbs are often considered what the body needs for energy. Glucose is the easiest form of sugar that the body can break down, and the easiest form of energy it can use. However, if you deprive your body of carbs or glucose, you can make it burn fat for energy instead. When you burn fat for energy instead of carbs, your body enters what is called "Ketosis". Ergo, the Keto Diet.

When you eat fat and carbs, your body automatically starts to use the carbs as its main source of energy. This is because carbs are easy to break down into glucose and be used for energy. When your body uses glucose for energy, your fat energy automatically gets stored to be used later by insulin. It becomes difficult to burn that stored fat because you're always refilling your bloodstream with more glucose.

Your body will always go for the easiest way to fuel you, regardless of what other fuel you're giving it. By reducing carbs, and instead of feeding your body fats, you're taking control of what energy you want your body to be using. You're forcing your body to switch to burning fats rather than carbs after it starves itself of glucose.

Carbs are often hailed as the best kind of fuel for your body, but that isn't true. You can only store about 2,500 calories worth of carbs in your body. But you can store up to 30,000 calories worth of fat! That is a huge amount of energy, and imagine the number of things you can do with it.

When your body makes the switch, you'll be putting it into a state of Ketosis. You've probably already been in a state of Ketosis after not eating for a few hours, like when you sleep. Ketosis is the state of when your body makes the transition from burning glucose to burning your fat cells. You start to make ketones after about 12 hours of not having any sugar or carbs. This effectively puts your body into a state of Ketosis.

It a completely natural metabolic process when the body does not have enough glucose for energy, leading it to burn fat in its place. Very simple, very natural, and very good for you. It can take a while for your body to get used to this, but eventually, you'll end up feeling so much better because of it.

Types of Keto Diets

There are several different types of keto diets. This book will mostly refer to the standard keto diet. However, there are options out there, and it's about choosing the right option for you. All of these diets can help you lose weight, burn fat, and balance blood sugar levels. All of them have their benefits and objectives. It's really all about what you want. Here is a comprehensive list of all of them to help you figure out which one will work for you:

Standard Ketogenic Diet

The standard ketogenic diet is best for beginners. It's also good for anyone looking into losing body fat and those who suffer from insulin resistance. Daily macros would look like this:

Protein Intake: 0.8 grams per pound of lean body mass, adequate

Carb Intake: 20 to 50 every day, 5% total calories, low

Fat Intake: 70% to 75% of total calories

Anyone who is just starting out with the keto diet should stick to this one before looking into other options. You might find yourself struggling with just how restrictive the diet is and will want to get used to Ketosis before switching over. Even then, you should only switch over if you feel like it's the right choice for you.

High-Protein Ketogenic Diet

If your goal is to build extra muscle and you've already tried and enjoyed the effects of the keto diet, consider this one. It's great for bodybuilders, weightlifters, and athletes—the people who need larger amounts of protein in their diet and need to build more muscle and get stronger. This is what their daily macros would look like:

Protein Intake: 35% of calories

Carb Intake: 5% of calories

Fat Intake: 60% of calories

Cyclical Ketogenic Diet

The cyclical ketogenic diet involves eating keto and low carbs for five to six days out of the week and then spending that remaining one or two days eating a high amount of carbs. It's good for bodybuilders and other athletes to maximize fat loss while building lean mass. Don't pick this one if you find yourself needing a bit of a break. It doesn't permit you to eat as much chocolate as you'd like. You still have to be eating healthy carbs.

Five to Six Days Keto Macros:

Protein Intake: 20% to 25% of calories

Carb Intakes: 5% of calories

Fat Intake: 70% to 75% of calories

Two to One Day Carb-Loading Macros:

Protein Intake: 20% to 25% of calories

Carb Intake: 70% of calories

Fat Intake: 5% to 10% of calories

Targeted Ketogenic Diet

The targeted ketogenic diet is where you target carb consumption around your workouts, a hybrid between the standard keto diet and the cyclical keto diet. It allows you to train at higher intensities at the gym and is a great option for people who are looking to maintain a high exercise performance. You eat on a regular keto diet the majority of the time, but all of your carbs are eating around your workout. Usually, about 20 to 50 grams total, before and after.

If you're already on a typical keto diet, it might be worth it to make the switch if you're looking to build up some muscle or if you find yourself struggling with your workout routine.

There is no straightforward answer for what kind of keto diet you should be on. Everyone is different. When you're just starting off, you should be trying different things, keeping track of what works and what doesn't, and paying attention to your body. Keeping track of things in something like a fitness app will help.

The Truth about Carbs

Carbs have gotten a very bad rap in these modern diet times. You're told, over and over again, that you must stop eating carbs if you ever want to lose weight, get healthier, or look better. Or you can't eat them unless you work out, or keep them contained in one meal, etc. Well, in rebuttal to this, anyone who follows a keto diet correctly understands that carbs are a must in any healthy diet, even if it's just a little bit.

Carbs are actually needed in your diet. They're one of the three essential macronutrients, along with protein and fat. So, what's the problem?

Well, we eat too many of them. Plus, most of the carbs we do eat come from unhealthy sources, such as fast food, starchy vegetables, and huge serving sizes. Too many carbs affect your blood sugar dramatically, leading to a risk of diabetes, constipation, atherosclerosis (a condition that causes disruptions in the bloodstream, leading to heart attacks) and vascular diseases. The biggest issue with carbs isn't the fact that we eat them; we eat too many of them, and when we do, they're not the carbs we should be eating.

This is why even if you decide that the keto diet isn't right for you, seriously consider looking at the number of carbs you are consuming. If your goal is to lose weight, remember: any carbs that are not needed by your body are automatically stored as body fat.

What Makes Us Fat

It is somewhat weird. It's called fat, but it doesn't make us fat. This made sense years ago when we just assumed that the fat in our food was causing the fat around our middles. It just added up. This started the whole "no fat added" campaign, which didn't help. If something says "low fat," this is basically just a label saying "there is a ton of refined sugar and carbs in this." So, stay away!

Healthy fats, such as what is in avocados, olive oil, and nuts, actually help you. They work to process all the food we're putting into our bodies, and our brains are actually 60% fat, so it's good for it too. Fats are very complex (which is why there is an entire chapter in this book devoted to them).

So what does make us fat? Well, this goes back to the sugar and carbs. If you eat more than what you need, they will be transformed into fat cells and put into "storage". This is the same with any food you eat. If you eat more than what you need, or over your calorie quota, you will gain weight. That's just how it is.

Mythbusting with the Keto Diet

The keto diet has gotten a lot of flak in the past few years. Many people have brushed it aside, assuming that it's just another fad diet. Of course, we know by now that it's not and that it will be around for years yet as a great way to lose weight and get your health back on track.

The Keto diet has numerous misconceptions and myths surrounding it, some of which you may have bought into. You should never go into a diet not knowing what is true, and what isn't true. You need to be well informed with the solid facts. Here are some of them, and the truth:

Myth 1: You can eat as much fat as you want, and it doesn't matter what kind you fill your plate with.

As much as we all wish there were a diet out there where you could pile your plate full of bacon and cheese without having to worry, the keto diet is not it. Until science gets there, we can just dream, and be realistic. No, **the keto diet's focus is on unsaturated fats.** Foods full of heart-and-blood healthy unsaturated fats such as avocados, nuts, olive oil, and fish, rather than saturated fats like cake, cooking margarine, and fatty cuts of meat like beef and pork. Even if all you're eating are unsaturated fats, you should be sticking to calorie counting and serving sizes. Calories are still calories, and too many will make you gain weight.

Myth 2: You can go on and off it no problem. It's a temporary thing, and you don't have to worry about gaining the weight back. It will stay off without any effort. Nope. Inconsistency with the keto diet will not just make you gain all the weight back; you won't experience the full value of Ketosis.

There have been reports of people who just do it for a few weeks before going back to their original diet, or even less time. This won't keep your weight off, and you will have an even harder time reaching that state of Ketosis.

Myth 3: The Keto diet is high on protein.

The Keto diet is not a high protein diet. **Protein should be eaten in moderation and kept careful track of using a scale.** Excess protein is converted into glucose which spikes your blood sugar. It also can lead to increased ketones, which sounds good, but can be problematic if you already have a high level in your body. Every person's protein intake is different and takes many things into consideration, such as exercise level, weight, sex, and age. If you're an athlete, for example, you'll need a higher protein intake than someone who only exercises moderately.

Myth 4: The amount of carbs a person needs is always the same, no matter the person.

People make the mistake of not knowing how many carbs are involved in a keto diet, or they don't understand just how little carbs it requires. On average, it's only about 20 to 50 grams of carbohydrates a day, which really isn't very much. To put that in perspective, a cup of spaghetti, cooked, without any added salt, is 43.3 grams of carbs. A medium apple, fresh with skin, is about 19 grams of carbs. The amount of carbs that you need during the day depends on the person. **Depending on your lifestyle, you may be able to go higher**. If you're unsure, make an appointment with a dietician or nutritionist who will be able to help you calculate what you need.

Myth 5: Veggies and fruit are high in carbs. You can't eat them.

Only do this if you have a desire for constipation, which can be a nasty keto side effect. **You need fiber**, and veggies and fruits are some of the best sources of it. They also have a ton of vitamins and minerals and antioxidants that are great for your body. The reality is: there are not a whole lot of food types out there that are completely free of carbs. You'll be hard pressed to find them, and the only things that will be completely carb free are oils, butter, and meats. Stick to veggies that aren't starchy (think potatoes and yams), and vegetables like broccoli, spinach, cauliflower, and zucchini. If you need sweetness, go for berries like raspberries and blueberries. There are plenty of awesome ways to make these ingredients delicious.

Myth 6: When you go on the keto diet, your body goes into ketoacidosis.

Ketoacidosis refers to diabetic ketoacidosis and is a condition related to Type 1 diabetes. People often get this and **Ketosis, the state that your body goes into when you go on the keto diet**, mixed up. Ketoacidosis is life-threatening, can develop in as little as 24 hours, and occurs when the body does not get enough insulin. Often when people hear the word "Ketosis", they immediately think "ketoacidosis". If people ask, be sure to explain the difference.

Myth 7: The keto diet by itself will help you lose weight.

People often go on the keto diet for this reason. Maybe it's the reason you picked up this book. The reality is: **there is no such thing as a diet that will automatically work for everyone**. Success in losing weight, and putting your health back on track, can and probably will be a long journey. It involves being consistent with an eating plan. People have different blood sugar responses to different foods. To figure out an eating plan that will work for you, please visit a nutritionist or dietician.

Why Should You Do the Keto Diet

The keto diet is great for weight loss, but it also has a host of other benefits. When you run your body on fats rather than carbs, your blood sugar will be more stable. You'll have a lower risk of diseases like heart problems and Type 2 diabetes. It will help cool inflammation in your body and reverse conditions such as a fatty liver and Metabolic Syndrome (a cluster of conditions: increased blood pressure, high blood sugar, excess body fat around the waist). Overall, you'll feel better.

Now, the question really is: should you do the keto diet? The keto diet will only work the way you want it to work for certain people. It all depends on your body. Genetics, body weight, age, gender—these things can all have an impact on your results.

The truth is that in the days of the cavemen, our diet would've been similar to a keto one. Lots of veggies, protein, and very few carbs—mostly because a lot of the carbs we eat today didn't exist. Our focus would've been on food that we needed to keep us healthy and full and strong, not on foods that would send our blood sugars spiking.

You should also keep in mind that some people should not do the keto diet for health reasons, as they might have a condition that will only worsen if they do, and it could be catastrophic for their health. This is why you should always check with a doctor before you embark on any big change in your diet, keto or otherwise. You should not try the keto diet if you have one of the following conditions:

- Carnitine deficiency (primary)
- Carnitine palmitoyltransferase (CPT) I or II deficiency
- Carnitine translocase deficiency
- Beta-oxidation defects
- Mitochondrial 3-hydroxy-3-methylglutaryl-CoA synthase (mHMGS) deficiency
- Medium-chain acyl dehydrogenase deficiency (MCAD)
- Long-chain acyl dehydrogenase deficiency (LCAD)
- Short-chain acyl dehydrogenase deficiency (SCAD)
- Long-chain 3-hydroxyacyl-CoA deficiency
- Medium-chain 3-hydroxyacyl-CoA deficiency
- Pyruvate carboxylase deficiency
- Porphyria

If you have any of these conditions, except for porphyria, they are usually identified early on in someone's life. Porphyria can be identified later on. If you have one of these conditions, you'll likely already know. However, you still should check with your doctor.

You should also ask your doctor's advice on the keto diet if your medical history, including your family history, includes any of the following conditions:
- Kidney Failure
- Pancreatitis
- Abdominal Tumors
- Gastric Bypass Surgery
- Gallbladder Disease
- Poor Nutritional Status
- Impaired Liver Function
- Impaired Fat Digestion
- Pregnancy and/or lactation

Keep in mind that doctors are not trained in nutrition all that much. They're not experts on the subject. They're often taught that Ketosis is dangerous, and thus don't know all that much about it. In fact, many doctors might very well get "Ketosis" confused with "ketoacidosis". If you want to make sure that they know this distinction, take this book to show them.

It is because of this that you should really consider seeing a trained nutritionist or dietician. They're specifically taught to figure out what people should eat and can explain to you what effect different foods will have on your body. A good one will be able to walk you through everything you need to know and tailor something specifically for your body. They will also likely know all about Ketosis and have easy plans on how to get you into it. There is a handy guide below if you do plan on visiting one.

Also, one last thing to keep in mind: a keto diet must be done right, no exceptions. In this book, we'll be taking you through every step of the way. So don't let yourself worry about whether or not you're messing up. You got this.

Common Mistakes Keto Beginners Make

We all make mistakes. It's part of life. However, avoiding them is a much more preferred option, especially when it comes to things like your body and its health. Thankfully, the keto diet, despite being new, encompasses many people who have made the below mistakes and now you can learn from them. Read this list, and hopefully, you can avoid the derailments of your ketogenic journey.

Obsessing over your scale. If you're in this to gain weight, it can be easy to get attached to the number on the scale. You weigh yourself several times a day, you have the number written down in several different places, and you always have the number of pounds you have lost memorized.

The keto diet has a lot of great benefits, and one of these benefits is weight loss. People have reported losing up to ten pounds in their first *week*. This isn't what you should be focusing on, even if your goal is to lose weight. For one, scale numbers rarely give the whole picture. There will be a ton of progress that doesn't even show up on the scale (also keep in mind that if you're working out, you'll be gaining muscle, which weighs more than fat). If you really want to measure your progress, consider buying a cheap measuring tape for sewing (you can get them very inexpensively at dollar stores), and use that instead. This will tell you much more about what is happening to your body than your scale ever would, and you'll see the progress happening right before your very eyes.

Also, two, the number can make you feel as if you're not doing well. It can make you feel as if you're not improving at all, even if you are, and might have you feeling discouraged. Keeping track of your journey is great, but how about focusing on how great you feel? Focus on how you can walk up the stairs without getting winded and how your skin has never been so clear? These things might keep you more motivated than a stupid number ever could.

Not enough fats. The average person is not used to their diet being 70% fats. They often underestimate just how much it is, and just how many you need to consume in a day to enter Ketosis. If you're 140 pounds, and you want to maintain your weight, you'd be eating about 160 grams of fat per day. To put that into perspective, an avocado is about 30 grams of fat per one whole fruit. To get 160 grams of fat, you'd be eating about five and a half avocados per day. Crazy, right? (Also, to be clear, these numbers are very rough so please don't take them at face value. Please do your own macro measurements for your body and lifestyle.)

If you want to make sure you're getting enough fats, be sure to track things like macros and use an app to figure out where you can get more of the good stuff.

Not eating good fats. People often get saturated fats and unsaturated fats confused. The whole "no fat added" and "fat-free" epidemic has done nothing to help that. If you're eating all the bad fats all day (think anything with trans fats), you're not going to reach Ketosis. If you're getting all these good and healthy fats, like nuts, olive oil, and fish, you'll definitely benefit.

As long as you stick to foods that you know are real and wholesome, with nothing added that you don't know what it is, you should find yourself entering Ketosis. Just avoid anything that has the words "fat-free" on it.

Too much protein. This is a very common mistake for beginner ketogenic dieters. When entering Ketosis, or keeping your body in Ketosis, you only need a moderate amount of protein because your body is using fats for energy. You only really need protein for building and maintaining muscle mass, so you will probably find yourself needing much less than you expect.

Keep in mind that if you eat too much protein, especially too often, the protein in your body will go through a process called gluconeogenesis, a process where other nutrients other than carbs convert into glucose. This will knock you out of Ketosis, and you'll have to start over. This process is pretty slow, so you don't have to worry too much about it, but it's just something to remember—another good reminder as to why it's important to track macros.

Not meal planning. This is the biggest mistake that beginner dieters make. They assume that because they have the idea in their mind, they can just stay on track. Think of meal planning almost like a map that is telling you directly where to go. By planning and making your meals in advance, you're removing temptation that could throw you out of Ketosis and helping yourself avoid falling short of your daily macro needs. By meal planning, you're literally giving yourself all the options you need without any need to order food. This can also help you maintain what is working and discard what is not. Plus, it saves time that is spent in the kitchen. You also might be able to find some amazing meals out there that you never would've tried before!

If you're not into cooking at all, well, you're going to have a hard time with the keto diet unless you have a private chef. Get into cooking by keeping it simple. Just focus on nailing these daily macros and then you can figure out how to put grill marks on the chicken.

Looking for a quick fix. One of the worst things that modern advertising and branding have done for living a healthy lifestyle is constantly referring to them as "diets". Diets imply something temporary. It implies that once it's over, you can go back to doing the same kind of eating you were doing before. The keto diet, and any brand of healthy living, such as the Atkins diet, veganism, or going gluten-free, is a lifestyle. It's not something you can switch on for a few months then switch off. You'll just find yourself right back where you started.

You might find yourself getting on the keto diet, and get yourself obsessed. You're obsessed with the results, you're obsessed with how great you look and feel, and you're obsessed with how trim your waistline is. You keep at it because it feels awesome to be healthy and to live your best life. Others, on the other hand, may reach that magic number on the scale or the tape measure and figure that they're done. They don't need to measure calories anymore or focus on the ratio of carbs, fats, and protein in their diet. However, they always wind up where they started—addicted to sugar and bad carbs and struggling to wean themselves off them.

If you're just looking to drop some pounds and that's all you want, consider just removing sugar entirely from your diet. It will cause a healthy drop in weight, and as long as you stick to it, the weight will stay off.

Not Getting Enough Sleep. You need sleep. Seven to eight hours of it, preferably. Lack of sleep can cause slip-ups, and make you crave bad foods. It also makes you hungrier, and it's harder for you to stop eating. You crave unhealthy food and want nothing more than to dive right into a basket of fries for that quick sugar rush to get yourself through the day until bed. Sleep is critical to your mental and physical health, so get yourself enough of it.

Not Drinking Enough Water. Your body needs water. In adult men, it makes up about 60% of the body. In adult women, it makes up about 55%. Either way, that's more than half. Water flushes out toxins, regulates body temperature, and improves digestion. You need water, especially if before you got all of your liquids from carb loaded drinks, like soft drinks, orange juice, and vitamin water. If you really dislike the plain taste of water, consider adding slices of lemon. However, the taste does grow on you after a while.

Comparing Yourself to Other People. This goes hand in hand with not focusing too much on the scale. Yes, the keto diet does lead to weight loss, an easier time focusing and feeling better about life overall, but you might find yourself wondering why you aren't getting these same results as fast as others. Every person's body is different, in both big and small ways. Comparing yourself to others also leads to big insecurities on whether or not you're doing the right thing.

On the keto diet, there are often very similar outcomes; they just happen at different paces. Don't focus on everyone else's results. Focus on yours, and how great you're doing. Everything should be done at your pace, and everybody's journey is different.

Doing it alone. Nobody should ever have to do something completely alone. Having people help you on your journey, and give you the support that you want, cannot be replaced by anything. It's a great feeling knowing that people want this for you, just as much as you want this for you. Doing things by yourself is difficult. So let your friends and family know about this lifestyle change you are embarking on. You don't want them tempting you by offering food that the Ketosis diet can't support. Maybe one or two may want to join you on your journey! But let your friends and family know. There's a whole bunch of ideas and tips on how to build this support system in this book!

Visiting a Dietician (or a Nutritionist)

Taking the step of going and visiting a dietician is a big step. While visiting any doctor can be nerve-wracking, visiting a dietician can make someone especially nervous. After all, the definition of a dietician is someone who looks at your current diet and tells you what you should be changing. Yeah, not fun. We have a hard time telling our family doctor everything that's up (which is not a good thing, stop doing that), so it's even harder visiting someone we probably have never met before, and just telling them everything. It can be a great experience, though, where you learn about your body and what it needs to be healthy.

Visiting a dietician is a great way of educating yourself. With a dietician, you can figure out what you need to eat, when you need to eat, find new recipes, and learn about all the benefits that come with your diet. You can clarify ahead that you're interested in trying a keto diet, and they'll have a host of information for you right at their fingertips. They can be a great motivator and partner for you in this journey.

Visiting a dietician should not be a painful experience. It should be one of enlightenment, and you should walk out feeling like someone really just helped you. It can be a great experience working with a dietician. Keep that in mind as you go in. Here are some tips on how to approach it, and what you can do to make the process easier:

- Be open-minded and positive. Walking into their office, make sure you know that they might say some things you won't enjoy hearing. Like you are eating too many bad fats, or you're not getting enough fiber intake. They might give you some hard truths. Look on the bright side, and open your mind up to the idea that they are only telling you this because they want to help you.
- Don't lie! Many people feel embarrassed about their eating habits. You need to work past any shame you have because the only way a dietician can help you is if they know what you're putting into your body. Don't claim that you eat salads three times a week when, really, it's more like three times a year. A dietician is not there to judge you; they're there to help you.
- Keep a food journal for a few weeks leading up to it. Leading up to your meeting, for at least a week, keep an honest food journal. Don't lie. Again, do not lie. Make a note of everything you eat. This will be helpful to act as a roadmap for the dietician, telling exactly where you need to go and what you need to change.
- Have a list of any medication or supplements you are taking. If you're on any medications, whether they're prescribed or not, let them know. If you have any long-term or permanent conditions, like diabetes, let them know. It could affect your diet.
- Consider a list of foods that you like. Really love chocolate? Put it on the list. Love carrots but would rather eat a shoe than broccoli? Put it on the list. This way your dietitian will be able to help you find recipes that they know you will like. They want to make eating a fun and interesting

experience for you, not a chore. They don't want to fill your plate with foods you're going to hate eating.

- Understand that there is no such thing as one diet that works for everyone. Yes, we know that you're interested in the keto diet, but it may not be the one for you, thanks to health reasons. Or maybe your lifestyle. The keto diet doesn't always work for everyone, and that's OKAY. We're all different. That doesn't mean you shouldn't try, but just be aware that it may not work. Our society needs to drop this idea of there being one diet out there for the entire world. No. Everybody has different needs and will respond differently to different foods.
- Be clear about what goals you have. Go in knowing what you want. Is it to lose weight? Is it to look better? Is it to get healthier? Is it to sleep better? Is it to stop feeling sick all the time? Whatever your reasons are for trying the keto diet, or any other diet, make sure you know exactly what you want. You will have an easier time putting together and moving towards your goals.

Having a dietitian can be a wonderful support system. They only want to help you live your best and healthy life—remember that.

Okay, now that we've covered what Ketosis is, broken down some myths, and explained some stuff, now it's time to really get into Ketosis. Specifically, what makes Ketosis: ketones.

Chapter 2: Ketones

The making of ketones in your body is essential to any keto diet. The keto diet is all about encouraging the production of them in your body, before putting your body in a state of Ketosis. When you avoid carbs and sugar for about ten to 12 hours, your body automatically starts to make them.

Ketones are a molecule. They're water soluble, and a fuel source. They're derived from fat, and hold a lot of energy, almost like a small energy pack. Ketosis is when your body starts using them as an energy source. The adaptation takes time, especially as your body gets more and more used to it.

There are three types of ketones produced. Acetoacetate is created first, then beta-hydroxybutyric acid, which is created from acetoacetate, and acetone, which is a side product of acetoacetate.

Get Yourself into Ketosis

Yes, if you follow the guidelines for your diet set out in this book, you will find yourself eventually getting into Ketosis. Eating a low-carb diet will get you there—it's just a matter of time. However, there are times when you just want that push into it. Here are some things you can do to speed up the process:

1) *Coconut oil*. Coconut oil is all the rage these days. It is used on everything, from our hair to our skin. But there aren't that many people out there using coconut oil for what it was intended: cooking. Coconut oil contains fats called medium-chain triglycerides (MCT) which are absorbed very quickly and taken straight to the liver. They are immediately put to work, and converted into ketones and energy for you to burn. Implement coconut oil into your diet slowly. Go from one teaspoon per day to two to three tablespoons per day for about a week. You can use it for cooking, put it into recipes, you name it.

2) *More exercise*. Exercise is often about burning away these glycogen stores, and they'll always go first. They are your body's preferred source of energy, after all. The fewer glycogen stores, the faster you get into Ketosis. Pretty simple, right? Also, because it takes one to four weeks for your body to adjust to burning fats, physical performance might decrease for that period.

3) *Try a short fast or fat fast.* Quick note: your body has likely already been in a state of Ketosis. It often goes into Ketosis in between meals. When you burn away all your glucose/glycogen stores, your body feeds on its fat stores. Just consider putting yourself on a schedule of when you eat during the day. You could also consider a fat fast. A fat fast is where you go three to five days where you only eat 1,000 calories. 90% of these calories come from fat.

The quickest, easiest and most important healthiest way to enter Ketosis is to cut your carbs and up your fat intake. It will be difficult, and it may take some time, but it will be 100% worth it.

When you start producing ketones and getting into the state of Ketosis, there are a few ways of telling that you're there. Here's a list:

How To Know When You're In Ketosis

It can be a bit confusing as to whether or not you're even in Ketosis. If you're not sure, these signs are great ways to tell you if you're on track:

4) Bad breath. People often report bad breath following the ketone diet. It is caused by acetone and takes on a sweet, fruity smell. Ketogenic dieters brush their teeth more often and chew sugar-free gum. If you decide to chew gum, check for carbs on the nutrition label. For teeth brushers, consider getting a travel size and keep in your car or bag at all times.

5) Weight loss. At the beginning of a keto diet, you'll experience significant weight loss in a short amount of time. This is not fat being shed, but rather stored carbs and water. After the initial water drop, weight loss should occur consistently. This, of course, depends on you sticking to the diet and your calorie deficit.

6) Loss of appetite. Scientists are still unsure as to why this is, and more research is being done every day. One hypothesis is that it's due to increased protein and vegetable intake. On the keto diet, you're much more aware of what you're eating and are probably eating healthier than you did before. Because you're eating better, you're not as hungry anymore. It could also be the newly made ketones in your blood. They may be able to affect your brain and suppress your appetite.

7) Increased thirst. As the body starts repelling excess water, sodium, and carbs, you might find yourself peeing a lot. You also will find yourself very thirsty. Sip on water throughout the day to make yourself feel better.

8) Increased focus and more energy. Constantly being tired, feeling as if your brain is full of clouds, and feeling nauseous are all symptoms of the early stages of the keto diet. These issues often lead people to give up. After they get through this initial state, though, ketogenic dieters report more energy

and focus. Their mindset has become sharper. To get to this, your body must adapt to the changes in what it's getting for fuel. The ketones in your blood are helping your brain (which is 60% fat!) and making it work better. Ketones can also help with brain diseases and conditions, like concussions and memory loss. They can stabilize blood sugars, which could also help your brain.

9) Short-term tiredness. Being tired sucks. It especially sucks when it is your diet that is making you tired—when feeding your body should have the opposite effect. Tiredness is the biggest short-term issue for newly ketogenic dieters. It often causes people to give up. Who wants to be tired all the time? This is totally natural. Your body is adjusting to the fact that it's getting a new kind of fuel. It's like you're remaking your entire body's energy system, switching from one source to another. The majority of your body's energy is going to do that. This process can last anywhere from seven days to four weeks. To help yourself get through this, consider picking up some electrolyte supplements of sodium, magnesium, and potassium.

10) Short-term decrease in performance. Again, your body is used to running off one energy source. It has to adjust. This leads to tiredness, but also performance issues, at work and in exercise. The reduction of your glycogen stores, which up until now was your body's fuel source and the most efficient fuel source it has, leads to having to work harder to find these other fuel sources, such as your fat stores. It's like sore muscles; it needs to work at getting stronger, and as you do it more, it will get stronger. After several weeks, it will go to work again, and work better than it used to! You'll find yourself with more energy and the ability to do more than you used to.

11) Digestive system issues. The digestive system does not like change (at first). It gets used to what it's getting. It knows what to expect. By changing your diet, especially to

something like the keto diet, you're majorly changing what it gets. This leads to issues like constipation and diarrhea. They might subside after a few weeks, but be mindful of what you're eating. Make sure you're getting a ton of low-carb, full of fiber veggies. Don't let yourself eat the same thing over and over again, even if you're doing the keto diet. A diverse palate will not only keep you from getting bored but will also decrease risks of digestive issues and nutrient deficiencies.

12) Insomnia, or Restless Sleep. This is another thing that tends to happen in the first few weeks. Many people who first start the keto diet report that they can't fall asleep, or they wake up several times over the course of a night. This should improve after a few weeks. There are no studies as to why this is, but it might be because your body is working extra hard to digest and use the fuel you're giving your body.

If you find yourself with these symptoms, you're very likely in some form of Ketosis. If you're still unsure, think of it this way: as long as you're following guidelines and your diet, you should be in Ketosis. If you're losing weight, enjoying yourself, and feeling healthy, no need to worry.

However, if you still want to know then consider a scientific test.

Tests

Measuring the ketones in your body with medical tests can be very useful. It will help you figure out when you feel best, and what is working for you and what is not. Using tests to monitor your Ketosis level is popular among people who are using the ketogenic diet.

There are three individual tests: blood, urine, and breath. All of them have pros and cons, and it's up to you to decide which one works for you.

Blood tests are the most accurate. They measure the ketone level in your blood and can tell you where you are in your ketone level. On the downsides, they can be very expensive and involve pricking your finger for blood. If you're a squeamish person, you might not want to. But if you think you could get used to it, try it out.

Urine tests are inexpensive and widely available. They're easy to use, almost like a pregnancy test, and non-invasive. Unfortunately, they are much less accurate. Urine is a waste product, meaning it's flushing out all of the stuff in your system. If you have ketones in your urine, this means that they're unused and unneeded. As your body uses more ketones for energy, you'll have less in your urine.

The last option is a breath test. Similar to a breath test for alcohol, it's a small, one-time purchase device, and it's very easy to use. It's the newest technology, so it does have limited research. Similar to urine, it's much less accurate than blood. It measures acetone, which relates to low blood ketone levels.

Ketone Supplements

One option is to help put your body in a Ketosis state is to try ketone supplements, which are called exogenous ketones. This means they're not made inside your body—rather they come from an external source. They're made in a lab and put in supplement form for you to try them. You find them in health stores.

Sometimes maintaining a steady ketogenic state just isn't realistic. Maybe it's your lifestyle, or maybe you slipped off the rails for a bit on vacation with your family. Either or, sometimes people just can't do it all the time. This is why people often take supplements; they can be a huge help in pushing you into that Ketosis state. You can do it right away—rather than wait a few days for your body to slip into it.

There are several different kinds of ketone supplements. Some of them taste all right, but they often don't taste very good. Be aware of the fact that often products will be listed as a ketone product, but actually don't do anything. Raspberry ketones are a very popular product on the market, but they actually don't work. Unfortunately, you'll find these products often.

It's not a bad idea to do your own research into ketone products. Don't fall for any advertising claims, and don't put anything into your body if you don't know exactly what's in it, and how it will help you reach that state of Ketosis.

So, that's it. That's pretty much all the scientific stuff about Ketosis, without too much scientific mumbo jumbo thrown in there. Now you should've grasped what Ketosis and ketones are. However, you may still be on the fence as to whether or not you want to embrace ketones into your lifestyle. Seeing as we are going to talk about the benefits of the keto diet, we're also going to talk about one of the biggest drug epidemics hitting North America right now: sugar.

Chapter 3: Benefits of Ketosis

The biggest reason why many people look towards the keto diet is weight loss. They want to lose weight and look good for the beach next summer. They also want to feel better about themselves, and embrace the idea of being able to go through their day without worrying about how they look and how people feel. With a lot of diets, this is the only benefit they have.

People choosing their diet based only on weight loss can lead to poor choices. When looking for a diet, people almost always just focus on this benefit. Losing weight is a great thing, especially if it's something you work hard for. Things such as exercise and eating healthy are some of the easiest ways to prevent conditions like kidney failure and heart disease. However, you should lose weight in a way that is good for you and your body. Your diet should have more than just that one benefit.

One reason this is a bad benefit—if weight loss is the sole reason for why you've picked a certain diet—is that it's not sustainable. At the end of the day, you're eventually going to reach your weight loss goal. What else will keep you going after this? What will drive you to completely embrace the lifestyle so that you keep the weight off permanently? Diets only work long term if you keep going at them, long after you've reached your weight goal and continue on the healthy lifestyle you're now in.

This is what makes the keto diet different. Once you completely immerse yourself in a state of Ketosis, you're now experiencing a host of other benefits besides weight loss. You become addicted to all of the other amazing benefits, not just the weight loss. Things like more energy to run around, skin without any blemishes, and just in general feeling so much better about yourself and your body, regardless of how much weight you've lost.

The weight loss is pretty great. Nobody's saying otherwise. The keto diet comes with quite a bit of weight loss. In the first week, people report up to ten pounds lost. This isn't fat losses, to be clear; this is the excess water and carbs in your body getting shed and being used up for energy. After this initial weight loss, you should be losing about one to two pounds a week, which is usually the amount that is considered healthy. This is great, but there is a host of other benefits to the keto diet. After all, there's a reason why celebrities like Kourtney Kardashian and LeBron James have sung the diet's praises.

One of the biggest reasons that diets often fail is because of appetite control. It can be hard to resist foods that you've always enjoyed, especially if you're already hungry. We've all been super hungry and eaten way more than we were supposed to. Well, good news—the keto diet helps with appetite control. It helps you make better choices in how much you need, or what you need. There are people on the keto diet who find themselves trying intermittent fasting, where you eat at select times and the rest of the time you don't. This is all thanks to the fact that they're better able to focus and say no.

Speaking of focus, people on the keto diet have an easier time doing just that, in work, at home, and otherwise. Their work production levels are higher—being able to get things done rather than procrastinating. When you're fueling your body with carbs, you don't realize just how much they're affecting your focus and making your brain feel foggy. The reason? Carbs cause blood sugars to rise and fall like crazy, and the energy source is not a consistent wave of energy. Ketones, on the other hand, are a consistent and steady battery that won't run out so easily.

Your energy levels go up because your body can only store so much glycogen (what glucose turns into when it's stored). You need to be storing and refueling yourself with more constantly. Your body can store much more fat; ergo, can store more energy in the form of fats rather than carbs. Is this why many athletes have turned to the diet to help them get through the day feeling like 100 bucks.

By eliminating many sugars from your diet, you're also reversing any issues with your pancreas and insulin production, meaning you're no longer at risk for Type 2 Diabetes. Type 2 Diabetes is one of these conditions that is very preventable and is caused by eating so much sugar that your pancreas goes into overdrive production trying to take care of it all. The keto diet is the opposite of this.

Another great health benefit of the keto diet is that it increases cholesterol. Yes, you may be panicking at reading that word as it's often associated with bad things, but we're not talking about that cholesterol. Your body produces two kinds: good and bad. Good cholesterol is called HDL, which carries cholesterol to the liver, where it can be reused and/or extracted. LDL is the bad cholesterol, which carries cholesterol to the rest of the body. The keto diet encourages the good cholesterol and reduces the amount of bad cholesterol. This reduces the chance of heart problems.

Another thing that helps reduce the chance of heart problems is having low blood pressure, which is another side effect of the keto diet. High blood pressure is often caused by too many carbs and sodium in your diet, and can be detrimental to your health. Having a steady, well-adjusted blood pressure is good for you.

The keto diet has also shown to have health benefits for some health conditions. These include epilepsy, Type 2 Diabetes, metabolic syndrome, and more. There are still many studies going on looking more into this, but it's not a bad idea to talk to your doctor if you have this or any other health issue. Do your own research into whether or not it may help.

The effect of the keto diet isn't just internal; it's external too. Keto dieters prone to acne might find themselves with clearer skin. Thanks to the fact that they're no longer eating large amounts of sugar, carbs, and glucose, all of which have been linked to bad skin, your skin could very well clear up. You'll be more confident and won't fear waking up with a giant pimple on your forehead.

The Bad Effect of Too Much Sugar

The keto diet is a very restrictive diet. Nobody is denying that. If you want to follow it properly, you have to cut out many foods that you probably very much enjoy, like candy bars, white bread, and even some (but not all) alcoholic beverages. You find yourself looking at nutritional labels a whole lot more, and having to put things back on the shelf because, well, it's got too many carbs. Carbs break down into glucose the same way in the bloodstream, so having too much of them will have the same effects on your body. It's not fun to do so—at least for the first little while.

However, to be fair, most of the foods that you'll end up cutting out, most of which have high amounts of sugar and carbs (which just turn into glucose) in them, are probably foods that you should be cutting out anyway. Glucose, which is often listed as another word for sugar, is actually found on many labels of candy at the supermarket, often in the first few ingredients (when listing ingredients, they're always put in the order of how much there is). However, sugar is not just found in candy; it is also found in tomato sauce, granola, and canned soup—it's literally everywhere.

Eating sugar is not just about weight gain and teeth decay, both of which are the main thing that people worry about eating too much of it. It's practically just another form of smoking, the new smoking, per se. It changes the structure of our cells the same way that smoking does, and strains the entire body when we eat it. It's not just about weight gain; it hurts every part of our body.

Your brain responds to sugar the same way it would cocaine. When you eat sugar, the chemical levels relating to happiness, dopamine, and serotonin rise in your brain. Just like cocaine, you want more after you come down from the high. How many times have you eaten a cookie, and an hour later immediately wanted another cookie?

Other immediate effects after having sugar are your insulin spikes, trying to deal with all the excess glucose in your blood. This leads to an eventual sugar crash, where you may find yourself feeling moody and drained and tired. In fact, eating a lot of sugar will often lead to you feeling very tired. Your body is constantly sending out insulin to help break it down. Add this to the fact that you are not getting the nutrients you need to energize your body means that you're going to be tired from eating so much sugar.

Long term, sugar can, of course, lead to obesity. But it's much worse than that. Sugar can change your cell structure, leading to them being able to resist the normal effects of insulin. It is not really understood why this happens. Your pancreas struggles to keep up with and absorb all the glucose in your bloodstream. Eventually, it becomes unable to keep up, and your blood sugar levels go higher and higher. There is excess glucose in your bloodstream, and it leads to Type 2 Diabetes.

Your liver also feels it. A healthy liver is essential to living a long and healthy life. Your body needs it, and it has many functions. One of these is that it regulates the blood sugar in your body, and helps fill up your energy reserves. When you need energy for later, it releases the stores back into the bloodstream. It can only store so much, however, and a surplus of it will turn into fat deposits. This can lead to liver disease. Fatty liver disease, where your liver holds more fat than it can metabolize, can develop within five years and can happen even quicker based on dietary habits.

Finally, your arteries. Blood that is weighed down and saturated with sugar can cause huge damage to all of them. They can't handle the amount and think of your arteries like plumbing, and sugar like a huge amount of sludge. Your pipes are going to get tired pumping all that sludge. It can lead to heart disease, kidney failure, strokes, and a huge number of issues for yourself down the road.

Even if you choose not to pursue the keto diet, seriously consider lessening how much sugar you're putting in your body. Seriously, it could save your life.

The unfortunate part is that sugar is virtually everywhere. There are many foods (like tomato sauce) that have sugar in them, and you might not even know it. To cut down on your sugar intake, start looking at nutritional labels and cut out things like candy bars and soda. That's a good start.

The Truth about the "Dangers" of Low-Carb Diets

Right alongside the "no carb" movement, there came a slew of well-meaning health professionals protesting it. Article upon articles were published on how carbs are good for you, followed by a wave of research to prove it. Carbs aren't the problem, scientists insisted; it's the fact that we need to eat good carbs.

This is true. We need good carbs in our diet, and even in the keto diet, you're still getting some. We need the glycogen to repair muscles and do things like work out. No one is saying that you need to cut carbs out completely. There is a difference between no carbs and low carbs.

Unfortunately, a whole lot of studies have been published, all about how dangerous low-carb diets are. Most people take them at face value, read the headline, and stuff their faces full of carbs, way overdoing it. They get scared off from trying the ketogenic diet entirely. Well, you're going to want to hear this: they're full of hooey.

Most health professionals who steer people away from the ketogenic diet mean well, but they probably don't know that much about it. Like we covered earlier, of course, some people should not be on a diet at all. The majority, though, would benefit in terms of their health.

Many articles railing against the keto diet will often list its side effects, but the majority of them are temporary and manageable. Once your body becomes accustomed to being reliant on a new fuel source, they become a distant memory, and you don't have to worry anymore.

As for these scientific studies that show that a low-carb diet isn't good for you, well, look a little closer. Most of these studies consider a "low-carb diet" to be 40% of their participants' daily calorie intake. That is not a low-carb diet. Many people who follow low-carb diets would agree that 40% of your calories coming from carbs is a moderate-to-high intake. Researchers should really be basing their research on actual low-carb diets.

Usually, when scientists do choose to have a study based on an actual ketogenic diet, what do they use? Rats. They use rats. Rodents are not people, and it is baffling to see just how easily people are willing to swallow studies done on other creatures other than ourselves. People should not be eating based on the effects that ketogenic rat food has on mice, rats, and other rodents.

If you're really nervous about trying a ketogenic diet, after listing all the benefits, do your own research. Don't just look at the headlines. This is a problem in our society where we constantly take all our information from just that one sentence. Headlines can often be very misleading (this is mostly due to websites wanting to get more clicks, not a genuine desire to mislead people). If you want to look more into the studies of the risks of low-carb diets, read the studies and know what they did to get these results. You may learn something.

So we've covered pretty much all you need to know about the diet. We've covered the science, myths, benefits, and how low-carb diets are good for you. Now it's time to get started preparing for your journey. The first step to this? Figuring out your macro count.

Chapter 4: Macros

Calorie counting is considered a staple in nearly every single diet. Its baseline is pretty simple: you count the number of calories you eat, so you know where to stop or where to get to. By keeping track of your calories, you're knowing how much you're eating, and how much you need to eat to keep within your goals.

The keto diet is slightly different in that regard. With many diets, you really just need to focus on the calories. You don't have to worry too much about anything else if your only goal is to lose weight. In the keto diet, you also have to count macros as well. What are macros?

We already went over them a bit in Chapter 1, but macros are the three main nutrients that should make up every meal: carbohydrates, fats, and protein. In every healthy diet, you should be getting a certain amount of each of these. It's like how your mom told you growing up that you needed to fill half your plate with green veggies. That's actually pretty true.

The difference between the keto diet and just any old diet is that you really need to focus on these macros. Calories are important too, but macros are especially important. Now we're going to talk about them, and we're going to go over what their specific role is in our diet, and why they're important.

Carbs

Carbs are considered the bad guy in the keto diet, and ketogenic dieters put a lot of time and effort into avoiding them. But we can't avoid them completely, which is a big mistake that many beginner keto dieters make. We need carbs, whether we like it or not. We don't need nearly as many as we eat, but we still need them. Important bodily functions like our liver and our kidneys use glucose to fuel them so they can do their jobs, and even our brains need a little shot of glucose.

Another reason we can't quit carbs? Fiber. Fiber is essential to any healthy diet, and it goes hand in hand with carbs. Look at the nutritional label, and you'll see fiber right underneath carbohydrates. Fiber is incredibly important for our digestive health, helping us feel full and improves good cholesterol. For men, you need an average of about 30 grams a day, and for women 24 grams. Fiber also doesn't get counted the same as macros. This is because fiber isn't digested the same way most nutrients are. Instead, it's used and discarded. The fiber count in your diet won't count towards your overall carbs.

Picking what carbs will make up that 5% can be tricky, but soon it will be second nature. It's about being able to read nutrition labels and look at ingredient lists. Look for ingredients such as glucose, galactose, fructose, sucrose, lactose, and maltose. These are all forms of simple sugars often found on ingredient boxes, and the ones you should be avoiding. You want complex sugars, like starch, in your diet. Starch is found in many fruits and vegetables, and many of them are perfect for the keto diet.

There is a whole section next chapter about foods you can eat on the keto diet, but for now, think of leafy greens, legumes, and fruits. These are healthy examples of fiber, and good choices of carbs to eat. However, think of anything that is high in fiber, high in nutrients, and low calorie. If you stick to these rules, you should be fine.

Protein

If you're brand spanking new to the ketogenic diet, protein will be the one thing that won't have too much of a difference. Your intake will stay pretty much the same.

Protein is important because of how much it does for your body. It basically helps build a massive proportion of it, such as your hair and your nails, and behaves as the foundation for things like blood, bones, muscles, skin, and bone cartilage. Protein is also essential in the production of enzymes, hormones, and other body chemicals.

Protein is also needed for your body rebuilding itself when it's injured. It repairs sore muscles, reducing muscle loss, helping build lean muscle, and curb hunger. When you eat, it is thanks to protein that you will be feeling full.

Your body does not store protein the same way it does carbs and fats, which is why you need to keep up with eating it. After a hard workout, it will be the protein that will get your recovery moving faster. Picking healthy, plant-based or, otherwise, protein sources will help you feel good and like you can conquer the world.

Fats

With any keto diet, fats are where it's at. Out of all the macros, fats are the most calorically dense of all of them. There are about nine calories per gram of fat, while both other macros have an average of about four calories. This will, of course, depend on the food you are sourcing it from.

Fat is a reserve for energy storage in the body. In the days of cave dwellers, when there could be weeks between meals, it was used as an energy store to keep our ancestors going through the weeks. Believe it or not, several thousand years ago, it was considered attractive to be overweight and have a lot of fat stored away for these hard times. Fat is what provides us with a layer of insulation for our organs and keeping our body temperature up. Fat also plays an important role in our cellular and hormonal health and is one of the primary sources of energy for our brains. It keeps our skin soft and healthy.

Like we said before, fat does get a bad rap in the dieting world. The lie of the "zero fat" or "no fat" product has only strengthened it. Just stick to the healthy fats, and you'll be burning these ketones in no time.

Measuring Your Calories and Macros

Now that we know and understand macros, and the importance of protein, carbs, and fat, now it's time to measure how much of them we need. The basic guidelines of the keto diet, 75% fat, 20% protein, and 5% carbs are usually a rough estimate. It will depend on person to person, and even the calculations done here are only a ballpark rate.

It will be up to you to pay attention to your body, to figure out what's working and what isn't, depending on your goals. If you want to lose weight and it's not happening, you can adjust your calorie rate. If you're hoping to build up some muscle and lifting weights isn't getting any easier, you're going to have to up your protein intake. Paying attention to your body is essential to any healthy lifestyle.

Before you begin the keto diet, you need to calculate the following:
1) Basal Metabolic rate (BMR)
2) Your total energy expenditure
3) Know your body fat percentages and lean mass
4) Adjust your calorie intake for weight loss or weight gain (or skip this step entirely if this isn't one of your goals)
5) Calculate your carb intake
6) Calculate your protein intake
7) Calculate your fat intake

This may sound like a lot of math. You probably were not expecting that. However, this math is only a small part of your journey, and all of it can be done with a calculator. If you don't have one with you right now, there are apps for that. There are also many places online that will calculate the rate for you, but you might just want to do it yourself. All of the basic math equations are done below. The only numbers you'll really need are your body weight, your height, and your age.

Easy peasy.

Your Basal Metabolic Rate

The Basal Metabolic Rate, or BMR as we'll be referring to it from now on, is the number of calories your body needs to do what it needs to do. Things like breathing, sleeping, eating food—all the basic things that you do every day without thinking. Everything you do burns calories and the BMR is the magic number we need to do these things without it being a strain on the body. The more mass you have, the more calories you need.

You can't get an exact rate. You'll never get to know the precise number that you need. All you'll be able to get is a rough rate, and as long as you stick in the ballpark of this number, you should be fine. The closest formula that comes close is the Harris-Benedict equation. It's considered the best way to figure out your metabolic rate and is the equation many dieticians, doctors, and nutritionists use.

For Men: 66 + (6.2 × current weight in pounds) + (12.7 × height in inches) - (6.76 × age) = BMR

For Women: 65.1 + (4.35 × current weight in pounds) + (4.7 × height in inches) - (4.7 × age) = BMR

If you're on the metric system, you better go for the Mifflin-St. Jeor Formula. It will be much easier for you.

For Men: 10 × weight in kilograms + 6.25 × height in centimeters - 5 × age in years + 5 = BMR

For Women: 10 × weight in kilograms + 6.25 × height in centimeters - 5 × age in years + 161 = BMR

Again, all of these equations can be done on a calculator. The numbers will come from your age, weight, and height, and also be influenced by your gender. Why?

For your gender, men's and women's bodies have different compositions and different builds.

Age because muscle mass declines after you hit 30, and that means your BMR decreases as well.

Your height and body weight because the bigger you are, the more energy you need.

Your Total Daily Energy Expenditure

Your total daily energy expenditure (TDEE) is based on the amount of energy you're doing. At this point, it's a good idea to be realistic. Planning to exercise and actually exercising are two different things. We're going to talk more about exercise later, but for now, just base it on how much exercise you're currently doing—no shame if you're not doing any! That can always be changed later. None of these numbers are permanent. Just be honest with yourself. These numbers will not work if you lie.

Multiply these numbers by your BMR, depending on which category you fit into.

1.2 = little to no exercise

1.375 = light exercise, one-three days a week

1.55 = moderate exercise, three-five days a week

1.725 = hard exercise, six-seven days a week

1.9 = very intense exercise, seven days a week

If you have a career that is physically demanding, like construction or one that involves walking a lot like retail or restaurant work, take this into consideration.

Your Body Fat Percentage

Measuring your body fat percentage is how you know the amount of body fat you have. Anything left over is your lean body mass. It will help decipher how much protein you need to maintain or build your muscle mass. Muscle burns more calories than fat even when it's doing absolutely nothing.

Your fat percentages can be measured in several different ways. It will all depend on you, your budget, and what you're comfortable with.

DEXA Scan: this is the closest you'll get to an accurate body fat percentage. It's an X-ray experience that measures your bone mineral density. While it is the most accurate way, it is expensive and can be very time-consuming.

Skinfold Calipers: These are the easiest to get a hold of and the most recommended. They're easily available at any doctors and gyms. Just head up to the counter the next time you're there and ask. If for some reason they do not have them or don't offer the service, they are not too expensive online and are available at many different retailers. They're also an investment, so if you're someone who plans on measuring your body fat a lot, these are definitely something to look into.

Body measurements: This is not the most accurate reading, but it is generally easy and can be done at home. All you need is a measuring tape, and to measure the neck, waist, height, etc. It will give you a good estimate. Here's what you should do:

Height: make sure you're barefoot and standing up straight.

Neck: look ahead, relax your shoulders, but no hunching. If you're a man, the tape should be placed below your Adam's apple.

Waist: the tape needs to be placed around the waist, the narrowest part of the abdomen for women and at the belly button for men. The best result you'll get is if someone else does it for you and your arms hang at your side. Breathe in and exhale slowly, and measure after you release the breath.

Hips: they should be measured at the widest part of the hip or butt.

You're going to get your most accurate measurements if someone else does it for you. It should also be done in the morning before breakfast. If you want to get a very accurate number, you could do it a few days in a row and choose the average.

Once you have gotten these measurements, head on over to the internet and look for a "body fat calculator". It's also called the Navy Body Fat Calculator. There are many different ones to try. Type in these numbers, and they'll give you your body fat percentage.

Eye it: Again, this is not going to be the exact, accurate number. Body fat percentages can be eyed—you just need a mirror and a bathing suit.

Look at our guide.

Stand in front of a mirror with your shirt off. Eye your abdomen, turn around and look at your butt, then your face. Consult the list below to find which one matches you best.

Men

Men have a lower body percentage than woman do, and carry most of their fat around their abdomen.

5% to 9%: this is not sustainable or considered healthy for most men. At this percentage, every single muscle is showing, with very little to no confusion, and veins are visible and clear. You'll often find this body in bodybuilders at the peak of the competition season.

10% to 14%: this is the body that people think of when they think "beach body" and is the body most men will strive for. There is a clear separation between muscles, but not all of them. Veins will show mostly in the arms and the legs.

15% to 19%: this look is very lean. There is little definition of the muscles and almost no clear separation between them. It is nearly nonexistent.

20% to 24%: this is the average body that the majority of men have. The separation between the muscles is not at all there, and there is a bit of fat around the stomach. However, it is not rounded.

25% to 29%: anywhere above this is considered obese. The waist is bigger, and the stomach starts rounding out. There may be a little neck fat.

30% to 34%: the fat has distributed more around the body. The waist is large around the hips.

35% to 39%: the stomach will have a clear protrusion and hang. It will grow over 40 inches.

Women

Women, as a rule, have a higher body fat percentage than men do. They carry more fat in their breasts, thighs, and butt.

10% to 14%: usually found in bodybuilders at the peak of competition and is not sustainable or healthy for long periods. The less vascularity, the father from 10%.

15 % to 19%: this percentage is usually found in fitness and bikini models. There is less shape to the hips, thighs, and butts because of the lack of body fat. There is little clear definition of muscles in the arms and legs, along with some visible veins.

20% to 24%: There is less separation of the muscles, and the majority of female athletes fall into this range. You're considered highly fit, and this is usually the body that women wish they had. There will be less definition in the arms and legs, with most of it in the abdominal muscles.

25% to 29%: the average woman falls into this range. Curves form around hips, and there is more fat in the thighs and the butt.

30% to 34%: there is more fat in the hips, butt, and thighs. They will be more rounded and pronounced.

35% to 39%: the face and the neck starts to gain fat, and the waist will be over 32 inches. The belly will often start rounding out.

40% to 44%: the thighs and the hips become very large, and the waist will be typically 35 inches.

45% to 50%: the waist will be over 35 inches, and the hips will be wider than the shoulders. The skin often loses its smoothness and will likely dimple.

When you've finally determined your body fat percentage, you can use this to figure out your lean body mass.

Body weight in pounds × point percentage (ex; if your body fat percentage is 25 then it will be .25) = pounds of body fat.

To figure out your body lean mass, take the pounds of body fat and subtract it from your original body weight. That is your lean body mass, and you can use it to figure out how much protein you need. You can also use the above information to decide what your goal is, and where you want to be in your fat loss journey.

Adjusting Your Calorie Intake

If you're not looking to lose weight, skip this step.

The idea is to eat fewer calories than you are eating to maintain your current, at this very moment, weight. For just starting off, take off only about 10% to 20% of your intake. If you wish, you may take off more, but you might find that it's harder to keep within that range. It's also not recommended to take off more than 30% for a long period.

To get this number, do this equation below:

(TDEE × point whatever percentage, if you're talking of 10%, it will be .10) - original calorie count = amount of calories to eat every day.

If you wish to gain muscle, you will need a few more calories. A 5% to 10% increase will help but remember: it will only work if you work out as well.

(Calorie expenditure × .05) + calorie expenditure = calorie surplus

Calorie counting can be tough, especially if you're not used to it. There are several apps out there that are designed to help people do this, and there will be some tips later on regarding how to make it as easy as it can be. However, good news—counting macros is considered more important than counting calories in the keto diet.

Carb Intake

You already know now that the keto diet is a low-carb one. You've already been told that 5% is generally the average amount of calories you will be getting from carbs, but it's really up to you to decide. If you want to put yourself into Ketosis as soon as possible, go for the 5%. If you want to work your way down, gradually cutting out carbs until you hit that 5%, do that. Some people choose to have 10% be their number. It's really up to you.

Most people need about 20 to 50 grams per day. Remember: your total net carbs will equal your total carb count minus the amount of fiber you consume. To calculate this:

TDEE × the percentage of calories you've decided ÷ 4 = the number of carbs in grams you should be eating per day

As long as you keep your carb levels in the 5% to 10% range, you should be able to get into Ketosis no problem. However, if you find yourself struggling to enter the sweet spot where you start to burn fat, consider lowering your carb intake.

Keep this in mind: when counting carbs, there is a difference between counting carbs and counting net carbs. Net carbs are basically the grams of total carbs in a food, minus the fiber. Fiber does not get absorbed by the body in the same way that other nutrients do, meaning that it doesn't raise your blood sugar levels or trigger insulin. So, when you do count your carbs for the day, make sure to subtract the carbs caused by fiber.

Protein

Protein should make up about 20% to 25% of your calories in the average, standard ketogenic diet. If you're having a difficult time entering Ketosis, too much protein may very well be the problem. This is a common mistake for beginners.

If you're not someone who is active, .6 to .8 grams of protein per pound of lean mass every day will do it.

If you fall into the moderately - lightly active category, .8 to 1 gram protein per lean body mass pound every day is for you.

If you are working towards gaining muscle, increase that number to 1 to 1.2 grams per pound of lean body mass.

Once you've figured out how much protein you need, use this formula:

range × 4 = number of calories you need

For example, if you have a lean body mass of 130 pounds and you're not active, you'll need between 90 and 104 grams of protein per day. Multiply 90 by 4, and you get 360, which would be the number of calories you need.

Fats

Finally, we come to fats. Fats will make up whatever percentage is left over from the other two, but it's usually about 70% to 80% of your daily calorie count. Add the protein and carb percentage you've decided together, and subtract it from 100. That is what your fat needs.

People are often surprised at how much fat they need to consume in the keto diet but just remember: it will all be worth it in the end. The benefits will come pouring in, and you'll feel and look great.

There is no guarantee they will be 100% accurate, so don't worry too much about that. Don't let yourself go there. The goal here is to have a range number to work with. The first few steps to any new lifestyle or diet are to figure out what works for you along the way until you are fully accustomed to the idea.

Chapter 5: Nutrition

Nutrition is a big deal in the keto diet. It's not just about eating a lot of fat; it's about measuring just how much you're eating. Keeping track is very important, especially if you want to get into Ketosis as quickly as possible. Here is a list, along with their nutrition information, but keep in mind that you'll probably want to look at the foods' actual nutrition labels. This will give you an idea, but of course, the number will vary depending on the brand.

Meats

Meats are a staple food in keto, and you'll have them in many of your meals. Meats have no to very little carbs and contain many vitamins and nutrients you need, such as vitamin B, potassium, selenium, and zinc. It is also a valuable source of high-quality protein.

To get the most of the benefits of your cuts, stick to free-range and grass-fed. They contain more omega-3 fats and more antioxidants.

	Portion	Calories	Fat	Carbs	Protein

Chicken	3 oz. (85 g)	187	11 g	0 g	20 g
Pork	3 oz. (85 g)	202	12 g	0 g	22 g
Steak	3 oz. (85 g)	236	16 g	0 g	22 g
Ground Beef	3 oz. (85 g)	231	15 g	0 g	23 g
Lamb	3 oz. (85 g)	250	18 g	0 g	21 g
Bacon	3 slices	161	12 g	0.6 g	12 g
Ham	3 oz. (85 g)	118	5 g	1 g	19 g
Turkey	3 oz. (85 g)	161	6.3 g	0.1 g	24 g
Sausage	2 links	150	13 g	0.7 g	8.5 g
Meatballs	4 (medium)	324	25 g	9.1 g	16 g
Roast Beef	20 g	23	0.7 g	0 g	3.7 g

Fats and Oils

Many of the oils listed here are pure fat sources and will help decrease heart disease risks. They're high in antioxidants and are a great addition to drizzle over low-fat foods for a bit of an extra fat boost.

	Portion Size	Calories	Fats	Carbs	Protein
Butter	1 Tbsp.	102	12 g	0 g	0.1 g
Coconut Oil	1 Tbsp.	121	13 g	0 g	0 g
Olive Oil	1 Tbsp.	119	14 g	0 g	0 g
Ghee	1 Tbsp.	112	13 g	0 g	0 g
Lard	1 Tbsp.	115	13 g	0 g	0 g
Avocado Oil	1 Tbsp.	124	14 g	0 g	0 g

Vegetables

While there are admittedly many vegetables that don't make the keto cut, there are many that do. All of these veggies are low in calories and carbs, as well as high in dietary fiber. It's important to get a lot of fiber, as it helps your digestive system and makes you feel full. Veggies also have a huge amount of nutrients and prevent heart disease and many different cancers.

	Portion Size	Calories	Fat	Carbs	Protein
Cauliflower	1 Cup (1" pieces)	29	1 g	5 g	2 g

Cabbage	1 Cup (shredded)	35	0 g	8 g	2 g
Avocado	1 fruit	227	21 g	12 g	2.7 g
Broccoli	1 Cup (chopped)	55	1 g	11 g	4 g
Zucchini	1 Cup (sliced)	27	1 g	5 g	2 g
Peppers	1 Cup (chopped/sliced)	38	0 g	9 g	1 g
Eggplants	1 Cup (1" cubed)	35	0.2 g	8.6 g	1 g
Tomatoes	1 Cup (chopped/slice)	32	0.4	7 g	1.6 g
Asparagus	5 spears	17	0.2 g	3.1 g	1.8 g
Cucumber	1 Cup (slices)	16	0.1 g	3.8 g	0.7 g
Mushroom	1 Cup (slices)	44	0.7	8.3 g	3.4 g
Onion	1 (medium)	41	0 g	9.5 g	1.3 g

Spinach	1 Cup	41	0.5 g	6.8 g	5.3 g
Lettuce	2 Cups (shredded)	16	0 g	7.5 g	1.2 g
Green Beans	10 beans	22	0 g	5 g	1.2 g
Olives	10 olives	44	4 g	2.4 g	0 g
Celery	2 stalks	20	0 g	4.5 g	0.9 g

Dairy

Dairy is not only nutritious and delicious, but it also fits right into the keto diet. Lots of cheeses are low in carbs but high in fat, and they contain conjugated linoleic acid fat, which is linked to fat loss and improvements in body composition. Plain Greek yogurt and cottage cheese are high in protein and promote feelings of fullness.

	Serving Size	Calories	Fat	Carbs	Protein
Heavy Cream	1 Tbsp. (fluid)	51	5.4 g	0.4 g	0.4 g
Regular Cream Cheese	2 Tbsp.	102	10 g	1.6 g	2 g

Sour Cream	1 Tbsp.	24	2.3 g	0.6 g	0 g
Blue Cheese	1 cubic inch	60	5 g	0 g	3.6 g
Gouda	1 oz.	101	8 g	0.6 g	7.1 g
Parmesan	1 Tbsp.	21	1.4 g	0.7 g	1.4 g
Swiss Cheese	1 cubic inch	59	4.6 g	0 g	4 g
Mozzarella	1 slice (1 oz.)	85	6.3 g	0.6 g	6.3 g
Brie	1 oz.	95	7.8 g	0 g	5.9 g
Muenster	1 slice (1 oz.)	103	8.4 g	0 g	6.6 g
Monterey Jack	1 slice (1 oz.)	104	8.5 g	0 g	6.9 g
Cottage Cheese	1 cup	213	9.4 g	7.4 g	24 g
Colby	1 slice (1 oz.)	110	9 g	0.7 g	6.7 g
Provolone	1 slice (1 oz.)	98	7.5 g	0.6 g	7.2 g
Greek	1 Cup	134	1 g	8.2	23 g

Yogurt (Plain)				

Nuts and Seeds

Nuts and seeds are full of healthy fats and have low carbs, as well as being high in fiber. Eating them has a ton of benefits, like reduced risks of cancers and heart disease. They're a great snack to have on hand when these cravings hit you.

	Portion Size	Calories	Fat	Carbs	Protein
Almonds (raw)	10 nuts	77	6.8 g	2.7 g	2.7 g
Peanuts (raw)	10 nuts	59	5 g	2.1 g	2.4 g
Almond Butter	1 Tbsp.	98	8.9 g	3 g	3.4 g
Peanut Butter	1 Tbsp.	94	7.9 g	3.8 g	3.5 g
Macadamia Nuts	5 nuts	93	9.8 g	1.8 g	1 g
Pecans	10 nuts	103	11 g	2.1 g	1.4 g
Hazelnuts	10 nuts	88	8.5 g	2.3 g	2.1 g

| Walnuts | 5 nuts | 133 | 13 g | 2.8 g | 3.1 g |
| Sunflower Seeds | 1 Tbsp. | 44 | 4 g | 1.2 g | 1.5 g |

Seafood

Fish are great for the keto diet because they're full of fats and rich in vitamins and minerals, like potassium. The majority of seafood is carb free, with a few exceptions like clams and other shellfish, but they can still be enjoyed in moderation.

Fish is also high in omega-3 fats. Omega-3 fats help maintain lower insulin levels and increase insulin sensitivity, meaning it's better able to do its job. It also has been linked to lower risks of many diseases and improved mental health.

	Portion Size	Calories	Fat	Carbs	Protein
Salmon	3 oz. (85 g)	175	10 g	0 g	19 g
Snapper	3 oz. (85 g)	109	1.5 g	0 g	22 g
Trout	3 oz. (85 g)	162	7.2 g	0 g	23 g
Tuna (fresh)	3 oz. (85 g)	111	0.5 g	0 g	25 g
Cod	3 oz. (85 g)	89	0.7 g	0 g	19 g
Catfish	3 oz. (85 g)	122	6.1 g	0 g	16 g

Halibut	3 oz. (85 g)	94	1.4 g	0 g	19 g
Clams	5 (small)	70	0.9 g	2.4 g	12 g
Oysters	3 (medium)	122	3.5 g	7.4 g	14 g
Lobster	1	233	3.2 g	5.1 g	43 g
Crab	3 oz. (85 g)	71	0.6 g	0 g	15 g
Scallops	5	72	0.6 g	3.5 g	13 g
Mussels	3 oz. (85 g)	146	3.8 g	6.3 g	20 g

Berries

Berries are a great way to get some sweetness in your life, especially since most fruits are just too high in carbs to eat on the keto diet. They're full of antioxidants and tons of other good stuff. If you're someone with a sweet tooth, berries will be able to hit that spot that wants a candy bar.

	Portion Size	Calories	Fat	Carbs	Protein
Blueberries	1 Cup	84	0.5 g	21 g	1.1 g
Blueberries (Frozen)	1 Cup	79	1 g	19 g	0.7 g

Raspberry	1 Cup	64	0.8 g	15 g	1.5 g
Raspberry (Frozen)	1 Cup	73	0.9 g	17 g	1.7 g
Blackberries	1 Cup	62	0.7 g	14 g	2 g
Blackberries (Frozen)	1 Cup	90	0 g	22 g	2 g

Eggs

Eggs are not just a great option to include in a ketogenic breakfast, but also very healthy. When you eat eggs, make sure you eat the entire thing, including the yolk. The yolk has the most nutrients.

	Portion Size	Calories	Fat	Carbs	Protein
Egg (large)	1	72	4.8 g	0 g	6.3 g
Egg (medium)	1	63	4.2	0 g	5.5 g
Egg (small)	1	54	3.6 g	0 g	4.8

Sauces

Keep in mind that buying these store-bought sauces can be hit or miss. Some stores have "keto-friendly" options, which is not a bad thing to look for, but they're still pretty rare. It will really just be brand to brand. Just be sure to check these nutrient labels, and consider making some sauces at home.

	Serving Size	Calories	Fat	Carb	Protein
Caesar Dressing	1 Tbsp.	80	8.5 g	0.5 g	0 g
Ranch Dressing	1 Tbsp.	65	6.7 g	0.9 g	0 g
Alfredo Sauce	¼ Cup	269	25 g	3.9 g	7.1 g
Hot Sauce	1 Tsp.	1	0 g	0 g	0 g
Mayonnaise	1 Tbsp.	94	10 g	0 g	0 g

Drinks

Most issues with drinks, like coffee or tea, is all the stuff we add to them, such as sugar, sugary coffee creamers or any other kind of sweetener. And let's not forget there is always water.

	Serving Size	Calories	Fat	Carbs	Protein
Coffee	1 Cup (8 fl. oz.)	2	0 g	0 g	0 g

| Tea | 1 Cup (8 fl. oz.) | 2 | 0 g | 1 g | 0 g |

Seven-Day Meal Plan

Keep in mind that this does not have to be your "ride or die" strict meal plan. This is just a good example of what your first week on a diet will look like, and many weeks after. For the first week, you should be keeping your meals simple, built around the foods you love, without doing anything too crazy in the kitchen—especially if you're not well versed in cooking and only know the bare essentials. Think of this list as a guideline, not a hardcore "you must do it this way" meal plan.

Day 1

Breakfast: Eggs, scrambled, in butter or olive oil, on a bed of spinach or lettuce, topped with avocado

Snack: Nuts of your choice

Lunch: Spinach salad with salmon or chicken

Snack: Celery and pepper sticks, with guacamole for dipping

Dinner: Pork chop with mashed cauliflower and cabbage slaw

Day 2

Breakfast: Bulletproof coffee (coffee made with butter and oil, find the recipe below), with hard-boiled eggs

Snack: Nuts of your choice

Lunch: Tuna salad with tomatoes

Snack: Roast beef and sliced cheese roll-ups

Dinner: Zucchini or veggie noodles with meatballs, topped with cream sauce

Day 3

Breakfast: Cheese and veggie omelet with salsa on the side

Snack: Greek yogurt topped with crushed nuts of your choice

Lunch: Spinach salad with salmon or chicken

Snack: Smoothie made with almond milk, greens, almond butter, and protein powder

Dinner: Roasted chicken with sautéed greens and mushrooms

Day 4

Breakfast: Smoothie made with almond milk, greens of your choice, and nut butter of your choice, with berries

Snack: Two hard-boiled eggs

Lunch: Chicken on a bed of greens with your choice of cheese and veggies

Snack: Bell pepper slices with a side of sliced cheese

Dinner: Grilled shrimp topped with a butter sauce with a side of greens

Day 5

Breakfast: Fried eggs with bacon and a side of greens

Snack: Nuts of your choice with some berries of your choice

Lunch: Beef burger on a portobello mushroom or lettuce "bun" topped with avocado and a side of greens or salad

Snack: Celery sticks dipped in nut butter of your choice

Dinner: Baked chicken with broccoli and peppers, a side of cauliflower rice and with a sauce of your choice

Day 6

Breakfast: Baked eggs in avocado cups

Snack: Kale chips

Lunch: Tuna salad and tomatoes

Snack: Nuts of your choice

Dinner: Grilled steak with peppers and broccolini

Day 7

Breakfast: Eggs scrambled with veggies, topped with salsa

Snack: Dried seaweed strips and cheese

Lunch: Grilled chicken sandwich with a lettuce "bun" with a side of greens of your choice, topped with butter

Snack: Turkey jerky

Dinner: Broiled trout with butter and sautéed greens of your choice

Bulletproof Coffee

Bulletproof coffee is a great way to get a little extra fat in you to kick off your morning. You might have heard of it by its other names, such as keto coffee, fatty coffee, butter coffee, etc., but the gist of it is basically the same; it is coffee mixed with butter and oil. The extra fat helps satiety and curbs your cravings and will keep you from reaching for a huge breakfast. The mix of caffeine and the butter will give you an extra boost and help you more than just the caffeine would (you can use decaf if you wish).

The main oil in bulletproof coffee is usually MCT oil. MCT oil is the fastest absorbed oil and goes straight to the liver to be converted into ketones. MCT oil can be found online, but coconut oil is also a great substitution. If you don't have either of these, something like lard or ghee will also work. The best combination is about one part MCT oil/substitution to two parts butter.

If you're used to having sugar in your coffee, you can put other sweeteners in it, like cinnamon or a little bit of cocoa powder. A little bit of cinnamon is always a great addition to your coffee, but cocoa powder is better for you if you're only a diehard chocolate fan. It tends to be pretty bitter.

Directions:

1 Tbsp. MCT/Substitution

2 Tbsp. Butter

12 oz. coffee

Prepare coffee as you normally would. Pour the coffee, along with your other ingredients, in a blender. Blend on high for 30 seconds. Enjoy.

Calories: 320 Fat: 36 g Carbs: 0 g Protein: 0 g

Foods That Are Off Limits

- *Fruit*: apples, oranges, bananas, peaches, melons, pears, cherries, pineapples, grapefruit, plums, watermelon, etc.
- *Grains and Starches*: rice, oats, corn, barley, bulgur, buckwheat, quinoa, wheat, rye, corn, etc.
- *Grain Products*: cereal, bread, corn, oatmeal, flour, granola, popcorn, crackers, pizza, pasta
- *Low-Fat Dairy*: skim milk, skim cheese, fat-free yogurt, cream cheese
- *Root Vegetables*: carrots, yams, parsnips, turnips, beets, potatoes, sweet potatoes
- *Legume*s: kidney beans, black beans, navy beans, pinto beans, peas, chickpeas, soybeans, lentils
- *Sweeteners*: sugar, maple syrup, honey, agave syrup, Splenda, saccharin, Aspartame, corn syrup
- *Sweets*: candy, cookies, chocolate, cake, pies, tarts, pastries, pudding, custard, ice cream

- *Some Oils*: canola oil, peanut oil, soybean oil, grape seed oil, sesame oil, sunflower oil
- *Sweetened Drinks*: Juice, smoothies, soda, sweetened teas, and coffees
- *Sweetened Sauces and Dips*: ketchup, BBQ sauce, most tomato sauces, some salad dressings, and hot sauces

Keep in mind that many of the foods on this list are referring to their store-bought, prepackaged versions, especially with things like sauces. Tomato sauces from the store often have a ton of sugar in them, but ones made at home will depend on the recipe. Consider looking into making some things at home if you're not willing to give them up.

It may seem like this list is super long. And very restrictive. You might see several of your favorites and think "I definitely can't do this."

You can. You can do this. You absolutely, 100% can do this.

Instead of thinking of all the things you can't eat anymore, or at least must eat in very small quantities and very rarely, think of all the foods you can eat. There is an entire world of food and recipes out there, all of them delicious in their own way and all of them different. Cooking should be an adventure and something you enjoy.

Too often we see nutrition as something that is a chore. Taking care of your body, fueling your body with the energy it needs to really get to where it needs to be, that should be one of your greatest joys.

When you focus on your meals, really try to pick out foods that you love rather than foods you think you should have. Yes, giving your body nutrients is important, but you should be looking forward to your meals. Nobody wants to cook something and then not want to eat it. That sounds terrible.

Look at the list above. If there is something not on that list that you enjoy eating in some shape or form, well, that sounds a little crazy. Pick out the three ingredients from the list above, balancing the macros, and build a meal around them. Even throwing them all in a pan and swishing them around in some olive oil or butter counts.

If you're a beginner cook, stick to the three to five ingredient margins. Just focus on getting these macros right and learning about this journey. It won't be easy, but you'll get it done.

Easy Substitutions for Foods

When first switching over, it can definitely be a difficult road of trying to figure out how and what you can eat, and disappointing when you realize you're going to have to really cut out many foods you have probably enjoyed and are a large part of your diet, such as pasta, chips, and rice.

Thankfully, though, there are some substitutes out there that you can easily make staples of your diet, and, in many instances, taste better than their carb and sugar loaded alternatives, with more flavor and variety, on top of all their nutritional value.

Lettuce Leaves for Tortillas

Tortillas and tacos are awesome, but their shells are basically all carbs. Replace them with large lettuce leaves. The crunch is similar, and there is a massive cut in the calories you're consuming.

Cauliflower Rice for Rice

Rice is often at the center of several meals and is considered a staple in many households. It can be difficult to give it up. Cauliflower rice is a great alternative because it basically tastes the same, but the only issue is that the texture is much harder than regular rice. If you are picky about the texture of food, this may not be for you. All you have to do is grind it a bit in the food processor, but only for a few seconds as you don't want it to become all mashed up.

Almond Milk for Milk

Almond milk is not quite the same as regular milk. It doesn't have much creaminess, and you can especially notice that when you drink it plain. However, if you're drinking it in tea, mixing it into recipes, or eating it with cereal, you will hardly notice. There are generally two kinds of almond milk: sweetened and unsweetened. Always go for the unsweetened version. Almond milk can be made easily at home. All you need are almonds, water, and strainer cloth. Another almond substitution is almond flour.

Cauliflower Mash for Mashed Potatoes

Mashed potatoes are one of the biggest forms of comfort food in North America, and can be difficult to give up. It's a big part of family meals, especially holidays like Thanksgiving and Christmas. Mashed cauliflower, which is made pretty much the same way, looks like potatoes, has the same texture of potatoes, and even tastes the same. You can add whatever spices to it that you like, and butter or cheese is always a great addition. Yum!

Fathead Crust for Pizza Crust

Missing out on pizza can be a huge bummer for ketogenic dieters. Pizza is awesome. Pizza is delicious. Even bad pizza is good pizza. Unfortunately, it comes with a ton of carbs, and most of them are in the crusts. Fathead crust is a perfect alternative made from almond meal or flour, grated cheese (mozzarella works best), cream cheese, and an egg. This may be a bit time-consuming, but it's so good! And if you're a big pizza fan, well... it's totally worth getting that amazing pizza taste back.

Portobello Mushrooms for Burger Buns

Everybody loves a good burger. It's a staple in many restaurants and bars, and you'll often find a lot of them bragging that they have the best burger in town, the county, or the state. While you can eat many of the ingredients of a burger on the keto diet, you're missing one of the two most critical ingredients: the bun. Some people are OKAY with missing out on the bun, but for others, you just can't have a good burger without the burger bun. Portobello mushrooms are the perfect substitution for buns, with all the softness and consistency as a regular bun, with a punch more flavor. You won't even miss the white bread when you discover this substitute.

Veggie Noodles for Pasta

There are many people out there who have turned to alternative forms of pasta, and veggie pasta is one of them. Zucchini is the best and makes some beautiful, delicious noodles. There are two options for making veggie pasta: using a spiralizer, which might be stocked in a total cooking store, but also can be ordered online, or, if you're not looking to make the investment before you have tried them, you can cut them up very thinly using a knife or a cheese slicer side on your grater. Veggie pasta is not only better for you and has heaps more nutrients in it, but it's also more flavorful and makes you feel so much better after eating it—other than regular pasta which often makes you feel bloated and overstuffed.

Spaghetti Squash for Pasta

Spaghetti squash is not quite the same as the spaghetti, but it's still pretty delicious. There is a tiny hint of sweetness within it that you won't get from regular pasta and it tastes good with tomato sauce. It also comes with its own bowl and is cheap and easy to make.

Kale Chips for Potato Chips

Chips are basically just deep fried vegetables with a variety of spices sprinkled over them, so there is no reason why you can't do this with any other veggies with just an oven. Kale chips are great, mostly because they literally take 20 minutes to make, and you only need kale, salt, and olive oil. You can add a variety of spices as you wish, but just salt works too. All you have to do is remove the stems so you just get the leafy greens, spread them out on a baking tray, drizzle a tiny amount of olive oil (two teaspoons—you need only a little bit or the chips will be soggy, and if you need more add one drop at a time). Massage the oil into the leaves, and put them in the oven at 300 Fahrenheit for seven minutes before flipping them over and putting them in for another seven minutes. Voila! All the deliciousness of chips with none of the carby downsides!

Meal Prep for Beginners

One of the best steps you can take for any new lifestyle is preparing yourself for it. This involves laying out your workout clothing, organizing your bag so you can grab it easily and go to work, having a car ready and waiting for you every morning—anything.

Meal prep is a great way to prepare yourself for a new diet. Not only do you save money and time by knowing how much you're going to eat and having to avoid working through a mountain of dishes every night, but you'll also be able to fight cravings better and avoid the inevitable time when you start to crave something that you shouldn't.

Meal prep can be done in one of two ways: you cook all your meals altogether for the next few days, or you prep the ingredients so you can have variety in your meals. There are downsides and benefits to both, or you can do a combination of both.

Cooking all at once involves you putting all of your meals for the next four to five days in containers, separating them out. This method works great if you want to spend as little time in the kitchen as possible or you have a busy schedule. It can also be really valuable in that you only have to worry about counting macros the one time. You don't have to do the math every single night, but it can be tiresome to eat the same thing over and over again, though, and it can be easy to fall into a ritual of just eating the same meals over and over again. If this isn't something that you feel you can do, consider your other option.

By cooking just the ingredients, you can make a whole bunch of meals over the course of a week, and mix and match to make what you want. You do have to worry about counting the macros, though, again and again, and you might have to do more dishes.

Doing a combination of the two can be valuable as well. You can do all the meals that require more heavy cooking (think stir-fries, soups, casseroles) while all the meals that don't require too much effort can be prepared (think salad dressings, roasted veggies, chicken breasts, burgers).

To-do List

Now that you've got an idea of what you want to eat, and how your first few weeks will look according to the diet, now it's time to go over your kitchen. Hopefully, your kitchen will already have many of the items you will need to get started. It can be a bit of investment, but it's totally worth it.

- *Clear all cupboards out of carbs.* If you live with people who aren't looking into making the keto change, consider having cabinets specifically for your keto foods. If you live alone, or your family is right there with you, donate it to a local homeless shelter, or give it away.
- *Kitchen tools.* You probably already have things like saucepans and knives, but consider buying a scale. If you're looking to lose or gain weight, a scale is very useful. After a bit of time, you'll be able to eye it without too many issues. Also, a body scale can feel really encouraging (but if you don't want to focus on that number, don't focus on that number). For kitchenware, stick with simple, basic, what you need tools, like a few saucepans, one or two frying pans, a set of knives, a good cutting board, some wooden spoons, and a spatula. Make sure you also have the tools to clean your dishes in your kitchen like sponges, scrubbing tools, dish soap, and gloves.
- *Stock up on keto-friendly foods.* You'll definitely want to stock up on things like oils, condiments, frozen veggies, nuts, and meats in the freezer. These things are always good to have, and they're the kind of thing you wouldn't buy every week. Consider a plan for every week that you go through

your entire kitchen and make a list of all the things that you need to stock up on.

- *Ketosis testers.* There are three different options for how to test that you're in Ketosis, and there is information about them in Chapter 2. It's up to you to choose which one will work best for you, and they can be a valuable asset to your keto journey.

Now it's time to really get started. The next chapter will guide you through your first week on keto, and help you with the keto flu, one of the big side effects of just starting out, as well as helping you with sugar cravings.

Chapter 6: The Keto Flu

The first few weeks of the keto diet can be rough. There is not only a lot of change to your day-to-day lifestyle (especially if you're someone who eats a high carb diet and you're quite simply just not used to cooking for yourself), it can also feel pretty terrible thanks to the keto flu.

The keto flu is something you'll probably start feeling within the first few days of the diet. You may not feel it at all. Some people manage to smoothly transition from a regular diet to a low-carb diet without any problem whatsoever. You probably won't be one of them. It can feel very similar to the flu, ergo the name "keto flu".

Symptoms include vomiting, nausea, constipation, diarrhea, headaches, irritability, stomach pain, muscle soreness, muscle weakness, sleeping difficulty, sugar cravings, muscle cramps, dizziness, and poor concentration. Typically, the keto diet will last about a week, but symptoms can last up to a month. The worst will probably happen within these seven days. This can often make first-time keto dieters throw in the towel, but you need to push through—at least for the first seven days.

The first day you probably won't feel much. You will start feeling something by the end of it, however, probably in the middle of the night. You will probably have a hard time sleeping and have to pee a lot. The next day you might feel as if you should just stay in bed all day, and this feeling will worsen, then get better, over the course of about a week. When you've reached that final day, which is a great accomplishment, you might feel better, but because it all depends on the person, you might still be feeling the effects.

Why does this happen? Well, think of your body almost like a house. Your house needs renovation. A big one. The wiring and plumbing are bad, your walls are not insulated, the floorboards have holes, and it's just not a good house. The keto diet is now changing out all the floorboards, properly insulating the walls, and fixing the wiring and plumbing. This will take time, and for a while, you might be sleeping in your house without walls. You have to feel worse before you feel better.

You can reduce symptoms, thankfully. Some of these ways include:

- *Drink a lot of water.* The keto diet will rapidly shed water stores, and replacing these fluids can help you with symptoms such as fatigue, muscle cramping, and especially digestive issues like diarrhea and constipation.
- *Avoid strenuous exercise.* If you are someone who works out, or plans on implementing a workout routine with your new diet, hold off for the first week or two, or until you feel like the worst of the symptoms have passed. All of your body's energy is going towards remodeling your body, and it must adapt first. Consider very light exercise, like going on walks or trying out yoga.
- *Replace electrolytes.* As your levels of insulin decrease, your kidneys reduce and shed the number of electrolytes, such as sodium. Replace them with tablets, gel, or packs to be mixed in a drink. Just check the sugar content. They can be bought at local fitness stores or ordered online.
- *Get lots of sleep.* Sleep is essential if you want to be successful in any part of your life. You need a good amount of sleep. If you have issues sleeping, consider drinking lavender tea, turn off electronics like cell phones and tablets

about an hour before bed, or take a bath or shower. The hot water helps relax your muscles and makes you sleepy.

The keto flu can last several weeks, with the first week being the worst. The first week you might find yourself wanting to quit, but do your best to just push through it. You got this. You're totally up for it.

Don't forget to celebrate when you've reached that seventh week—and not with food. Consider letting yourself do something you've wanted to do for a while, like going to see a movie that you've wanted to see or splurging on concert tickets. Something that will get you up and moving and away from food is your best bet.

Sugar Cravings

Sugar cravings, or carb cravings, are a very common side effect of the keto diet. This isn't just the keto flu; even people who aren't on keto but who are cutting sugar out of their diet feel these effects.

The biggest issue with sugar is that it's mostly a habit. We're used to doing something, so we do it. We're used to having ice cream after dinner. We're used to letting go over the weekend and eating whatever we like. We're used to eating dessert whenever we're over at a friend's house. We're used to buying a sugary coffee drink on our way to work in the morning. When something is such a part of your routine without even thinking about it, you find yourself more used to the habit. You're not just craving the sugar; you're craving the habit.

We've already gone over the bad effects of sugar, but that's not enough. People still smoke cigarettes decades after it was proven just how terrible they are for you. Why? Because it's a habit, and something they're used to doing. You can know all the bad effects of sugar. You could have them be the lock screen of your phone, have them tattooed on the back of your hand, you name it, and yet you might still find yourself craving that candy bar. While, yes, you're craving the dopamine rush in your brain, you're also just used to the idea of going to eat that candy bar.

Now it's time to learn how to deal with it.

The best course of action when it comes to breaking a bad habit is to replace it with a better habit. Buy tea instead of hot chocolate. Reach for the salad rather than the French fries. It can be difficult to fight this impulse, especially if you're so used to giving in. These urges can be pretty powerful, and there is nobody here saying otherwise, or saying that you're bad for giving in to them. It's human nature to stick to the things we're used to, and we're comfortable with, and you're not a failure for feeling these urges. Here are some ideas of what to do when you get the urge for chocolate:

- *Eat protein.* Protein can help reduce sugar cravings and make you feel full. Even just a handful of nuts could really help. Just make sure not to overindulge and eat too many. They're pretty high in calories, and too much protein in your diet will convert to glucose.
- *Go for a walk instead.* Walking or any light exercise will help bring dopamine to the brain and reduce the cravings. Just take a spin around the block in the fresh air, and the sun will not only kick that craving to the curb, but it will also put you in a great mood.
- *Tell yourself, "Later."* By telling yourself this, you'll have something to look forward to. Put off getting sugar the same way you put off getting out of bed or doing the work that you know is due in two days.
- *Work your way down.* Many people want to jump right into the keto diet and think they can just sustain depriving themselves all at once. Consider working your way down from your sugar level, one step at a time, rather than cutting everything out at once. This will help you feel less deprived, and you won't find yourself feeling like you're missing out. You could start first by cutting out soda, then processed sugars like what is in candy, then replacing them with other

ideas. You could replace soda with water, a handful of candy with berries, a sweet coffee with bulletproof coffee. The choice is yours.

It will also be really, really helpful to identify your triggers early on. Are your triggers social? Do they occur walking past a certain gas station or grocery store? Are they at a certain time of day? Is it something you just do without thinking?

Identify your triggers, and work to change them. Instead of buying a candy bar at the checkout aisle, call your partner and ask if anything else is needed. Instead of heading to the vending machine for that two PM sugar crash, bring a snack from home.

Remember: the craving is temporary. And the pain that comes with it is temporary. However, the feelings of pride and awesomeness will stay with you forever. Plus, you know it's good for you.

Chapter 7: Exercising

When people picture themselves making better life choices, they often picture themselves eating better and then following this up with a lot of cardio and sit-ups. This, of course, can be a part of the ketogenic diet, but first, you need to change many of the ideas you probably have over exercise and dieting.

When the image of someone "dieting" springs to a person's mind, they often think of someone who is eating much less than average and following up this pitiful meal by working out for an hour. This model is not only unsustainable but ridiculous. We've already covered that the keto diet can be full of rich, enjoyable meals that will fuel your body and make you feel good. Exercise can be equally enriching.

Just in case you don't know, exercise is primarily fueled by glucose. When glucose is stored as glycogen, it is the glycogen stores that get burned when you do strenuous exercise. So, you may be wondering how exercising works on the keto diet, considering that you're switching your body over to burning fat.

Some people may read the fact that exercise burns glucose and think that exercise is impossible. Or that they shouldn't bother.

To be clear: you can get by without worrying about exercise. The majority of our health comes from what we eat, and as long as you're moving around a lot during the day in the form of walking and standing, you should be fine. Although, exercise does have its health benefits. It helps makes our bones stronger, enhances muscle growth and sustainability, and is good for the heart. So, implementing even just a light exercise routine is very beneficial.

There are four kinds of exercise you can do:

Aerobic: this is what is commonly known as cardio and is anything that's high intensity and lasts for over three minutes. It predominantly uses carbs as an energy source.

Anaerobic Exercise: this is what people consider interval training. It requires shorter bursts of energy, and carbs are once again its primary source of energy. Think of weight training or high cardio interval training.

Flexibility: this is anything that stretches your body. Think yoga, or after workout stretches. This kind of exercise is great for your joints, improving your muscle range of motion, and helps prevent injuries.

Stability: think balancing exercises and core training. It improves alignment, strengthens muscles, and helps control movements.

What energy is burned really depends on the intensity of your workout, but the gist of it is this:

Low-intensity: fat is used as energy

High-intensity: glycogen is used as energy

Pretty simple, right?

However, that does mean that you need to consume more carbs if you do more high-intensity workouts. It goes back to the fact that the more you work out, the more carbs you need. You're going to have to adjust the carbs based on your lifestyle.

If you exercise more than three times a week, consider looking into a different kind of ketogenic diet, specifically the Targeted Keto Diet.

We already talked a bit about it before, but the idea is that you eat all your carbs around the time you work out. Eat 15 g to 30 g of carbs right before and right after. This gives your muscles glycogen to help your muscles recover, and any extra glucose will be burned away by the workout.

For the first few weeks of the keto diet, exercise will be pretty hard on your body. This means that for this time, you're going to have to take it easy, like with walks and light yoga. The longer your body gets used to burning fats for energy, the better you will feel. You will find your exercise performance will increase after a few weeks.

In the beginning, focus on the diet first, rather than the exercise. Feeding your body with the proper nutrients it needs and letting it adapt to the different fuel source is more important, at first. After your body gets adjusted, you will find it much easier.

Chapter 8: Socializing

You can control your diet in the kitchen, but in other kitchens, not so much. Eating is an essential part of our social life. We have food at parties, when we go out with friends, at the movies, and there aren't very many social settings that don't call for a drink at the end of the night. Unfortunately, when you're on a restrictive diet, keto or otherwise, you find yourself very limited by your options of what you can eat. Not only that, but you're surrounded by temptation wherever you go.

However, you need to socialize and see your friends. That's just how humans work. We need to spend at least some of our time surrounded by people we love and who love us. We need to have mental stimulation from good conversation, laugh at our friend's jokes, and have some good-quality fun with the people in our lives. Even if you're introverted and claim to hate people, you would probably find yourself driven completely stir crazy if you went without talking to anyone real for a few weeks. We're social creatures to our core.

So, how do you get around this? Well, one option would be to just nix any involvement with your friends involving food. This will likely not work because food shapes our social lives. You and a lot of the people you consider close friends probably have the same tastes in restaurants you enjoy going to. The second option would be to take some of the advice you're about to read seriously.

Eating out in restaurants. As people's diets are becoming more and more varied, restaurants have to follow their lead, or they might find themselves fighting for a big enough customer base to keep them from going bankrupt. This is the big reason why many restaurants have vegan and vegetarian options now, and many of them also have gluten-free and dairy-free menus on request for those who have conditions that prohibit them from eating these foods. Whether or not a keto diet menu will join the list in the future, follow these tips until that blessed day finally dawns upon us:

1. *Tell your friends about your dietary needs beforehand.* It's like this: if you were completely gluten intolerant, like to the point where you could not eat gluten, you'd die if you did, you'd tell a friend that if you were going out to dinner with them, or if they were making you a meal. By telling your friends upfront about what you can and cannot eat, you can pick a restaurant together. If you want to make the process smoother, research the restaurants with keto-friendly options in the area. Having a list on hand in the note app on your phone will be especially useful for these times rather than you having to go through the local menus each time.

2. *Eliminate starch.* If the meal has large amounts of starch as a side dish, like potatoes, rice, or bread, the vast majority of restaurants have salads and roasted or tossed veggies as other options. If it's not listed on the menu, ask! Many restaurants, especially Italian and Mediterranean ones, have bread baskets in the middle; ask for it to be removed. If the meal comes with starch that you did not expect, eliminate it by either throwing it away or offering it to a friend. You can tell the restaurant you have dietary needs beforehand, and this will make the process easier for you.

3. *Add your own healthy fats.* Restaurant food is usually heavy on the carbs and the unhealthy fats, but rarely on the healthy fats. This, of course, depends on the restaurant, but this is a huge chunk of them. Add your own healthy fats by asking for extra butter and drizzling it over your meal. You can ask for olive oil and vinegar salad dressings and use them on a salad. A lot of restaurants prefer the more affordable canola oil, which is far less healthy than olive oil. Seasoned ketogenic dieters know they should always carry a tiny vial of olive oil somewhere on their person.

4. *Ask.* Restaurants should always be completely transparent about what they're putting in their food. They should have no problem answering whatever questions you might have, and if you request to see an ingredient list, that is your right. You have a right to know what is going into your body. Period. If they do seem to have an issue with you looking into their food, or behave like you're crazy, well, you can cross that restaurant off your list of places to go to.

5. *Eat a snack beforehand.* This is especially beneficial if you have a hard time resisting temptation when it's right in front of you, or if you plan to be out for a while. Keep a snack in your bag if you're going out and about with friends. This will help you to stop reaching for the French fries. Just a small bag of nuts and you'll be golden.

6. *Go easy on the alcohol.* While some alcohol is totally OKAY when you're going keto, others are not. Also, be honest. Once in your life you've probably got drunk and eaten your way through an entire pizza or a huge bag of Oreos (no judgment, we've all been there). Getting drunk can lead to you being much less careful about what you're putting in your body. Be careful.

7. *Choose drinks with care.* Water, sparkling water, coffee, tea—these can all be drunk without worry. There are also many carb friendly alcohol options. It may take some getting used to, but you'll get there.

8. *Keep an eye on sauces.* Sauces often have huge amounts of carbs and sugar in them, especially those that are served in restaurants. Remember: restaurants want you to come again, and they want you to enjoy their food. This often means that they pack a ton of carbs and sugar into it to make it as delicious as possible. This includes sauces. Safe bets usually include vinaigrette, mayo, and hollandaise sauce, but ask for an ingredient list if you're unsure.

9. *Rethink dessert.* If your friends are all ordering dessert, go for a cup of coffee or tea. Ask if the restaurant can make up a cup of berries drizzled in cream if you really want something sweet.

10. *Know when to cheat.* One small plate of French fries every few months is not going to ruin your diet. Knowing when (and how) to cheat can make the restrictions so much easier, and keep your head on straight. If you're visiting a friend in another city and you're visiting a bakery that claims it has the best chocolate cake in the world, a thin slice will not kill your ketosis—but it may open up the doors to cravings, so be warned.

Alcohol

Weirdly enough, alcohol doesn't have nutrition labels. This is because manufacturers argue that because technically alcohol isn't a food, and you don't drink it for nutritional purposes, this means that they don't need one. This can be frustrating for people wanting to stay inside their calorie range, but they still want to have a good time and drink and dance.

Alcohol is another part of the social experience. People love to drink. If the United States of America couldn't get rid of alcohol completely, it's probably not going to be going anywhere, at least not in our lifetimes. It's your choice whether or not you drink. Don't let anyone tell you otherwise.

On the keto diet, you can drink, just not as much as before, and like almost every other food group, your choices are much more limited. Also, you need less alcohol to get drunk, which is a pretty great benefit. However, be careful. Just assume that your tolerance level has gone down by about half until you're sure. Nobody really knows why this is, but the theory is because the liver is busy at work producing and maintaining ketone levels, and it's too busy to take care of the alcohol. There is less capacity to dilute it from the bloodstream.

Alcohol should be enjoyed in moderation, no matter what diet you're on. However, if you're someone who often drinks, as in one to three times a week, and you're not losing weight, consider cutting back on the drinking. It may very well be the culprit.

All of these drinks you'll be able to find at your local liquor store, and the majority, if not all, will be available at any restaurant with a liquor license:

- *Wine:* Dry wine can be enjoyed with little impact. In a regular glass of dry wine, there are about .5 grams of sugar, and a tiny amount of carb remains, all of which add up to about two carbs per glass. This amount of wine won't affect your diet much, especially if it's not done on the regular and is instead an occasional treat. Sweeter wine, however, can have upwards to four carbs per glass, while a glass of dessert wine can have five to six.
- *Beer:* Think of drinking beer similar to drinking liquid bread. Some of them have over 14 carbs in a single, 12-ounce bottle. While there are some light beer options out there, it may be best just to stay clear entirely. However, if you really can't resist, or

just want a couple of cold ones for a special occasion, keep this tip in mind: the darker the beer, the more carbs it has.

• *Hard liquor:* There are no carbs in any hard liquors. Not even vodka, which is made of potatoes. As long as you don't add anything like fruit juice or sugar-laden flavorings, you're good to drink as much as you want. You can also add diet sodas (in moderation, remember) to the drinks.

Here is a list of some drink suggestions, ordered from lowest carb intake to highest.

Drink	# of Carbohydrates
Whiskey	0
Dry Martini	0
Brandy	0
Tequila Shot	0
Vodka and Soda Water	0
Bloody Mary	0
Margarita	8
Cosmopolitan	13

Gin and Tonic	16
White Russian	17
Vodka and Orange Juice	28
Rum and Coke	39

• *Coolers:* You mean alcoholic sugar? You may know these things by another name, such as spirit coolers, cider, hard lemonade, wine coolers, the list goes on and on and on. Either way, these things are all packed with sugar and a whole busload of carbs. You might as well just be drinking sugar, so you're much better off to avoid them like the plague. As time passes, more and more sugar-free ones will enter the market, but until that day comes, stick to other drinks.

• Champagne: Don't worry, when you're celebrating your latest promotion or at a friend's wedding or birthday party, you can still toast and sip on the champagne without worrying about the issue on your diet. One glass contains about one gram of net carbs, so sip leisurely.

Activities to do With Friends (That Don't Involve Eating or Drinking)

Food may be a huge part of our social life, but it doesn't have to make up our entire social life. There are plenty of things you can do with friends and family that don't involve either of these things, and you can have loads of fun and create a bucket load of amazing memories without food being at the center of it all.

Your friends and family should be your biggest supporters, so they should understand that you can't eat at the restaurants you used to go to. Let them know what you want to do, and if they really want to see you, they'll make it work. You don't have to go get coffee and a donut every time you see each other—and maybe your friendship could use a little variety.

1. *Try a new restaurant.* Yes, this list is about things that don't involve eating, but think about it: if you find a restaurant that has keto-friendly recipes, it's near the one you usually go to, and your friend is down to try it, go for it. Finding new food to eat and trying new things is one of the great pleasures of life.

2. *Go for a hike.* There is most likely a few local hiking spots in your area that you have been meaning to do but never have for whatever reason. Do it now, and bring the gang. Just make sure to pack plenty of water and some healthy snacks, like nuts and dried meat, such as beef jerky.

3. *Ride around with some bikes.* If there is a local bike rental place, or you have your own bike that hasn't gotten any attention recently, hop on it and take a spin. It's great exercise, you'll get some fresh air, and you'll see a part of your city that you've never seen before. Get peddling; adventure awaits!

4. *Outdoor movie or concert.* Look into your local listings, or on Facebook (events are often posted there). Ask around to

see if any people know anything. There are plenty of free concerts, especially in the summer months.

5. *Visit the zoo or aquarium.* Visiting your local zoo or aquarium can be both an educative and fun experience. You can take silly pictures with the animals and often they do training shows. Grab a whole group of friends and go!

6. *Head to the beach.* Who doesn't love laying around in the sun all day in between beach volleyball and taking dips in the ocean? Plus, you can get in some great calorie burning at the beach, whether it's swimming, playing Frisbee, or even just walking on the sand.

7. *Have a craft night.* Have a night where you all get together and paint, or draw, or learn how to knit. You may all be terrible at it, and all of the crafts may come out looking awful, but you'll have a lot of fun, and you'll learn together.

8. *Take a class together.* Speaking of learning together, taking a class with a friend is always better than taking one alone. Look at your local rec center for classes for adults they're having, like painting, pottery, writing, or even something like book study or cooking. They may even have a class on keto cooking coming up!

9. *Camping.* If you'd just like to get away for a few days with your friends, away from the temptation of carbs, or even just want a few days away from the craziness and bustle of the city, it can be really valuable to enjoy the stillness of camping. You and your friends can hike, tell silly ghost stories around the campfire, and go on night walks (just be sure to bring a flashlight, and prepare yourself, so you don't attract bears).

10. *Try a fitness class.* If you're also looking to include fitness into your lifestyle and have a friend who's also into working out, find a fitness class that you both would enjoy. Your local rec center, YMCA, or gym will have them.

11. *Watch the sunset or sunrise.* This can go hand in hand with camping or going hiking. Either get up really early in

the morning or in the evening and watch the sunrise or sunset with a friend or a group. However, if you live somewhere where it's easy to watch the sunset or sunrise from your place (the roof of your apartment building, perhaps?) consider doing that. If you're blanking on where you can watch it, consider checking out a local community group on Facebook. Most cities have them.

12. *Visit a museum or art gallery.* It never hurts to learn a little bit more about history, your town, your state/province, or your country. Keep an eye on the announcements to see if they have upcoming exhibits. Check out your local art museum for a touch of culture in your life, and, of course, to look at beautiful paintings.

13. *Host a bonfire.* This may only work if you live outside of a city and have a backyard. And well, a lot of stuff to burn. But if you ever find yourself in one of these positions and want to burn stuff (like we all do at times), just do it.

14. *Host a video game tournament.* Really into gaming? Do you or a friend have a great video game console? Or maybe you just got a new game? Either way, get together and host a tournament. Winner gets to wear the gaming crown for the night!

15. *Host a movie night.* This is a great idea for big movie fans. All you really need to host a movie night in your apartment is a Netflix account (or a cheap Blu-ray or DVD player), and a TV. Snacks are optional. Consider going for themes, like romance, Pixar, or horror.

16. *Have them over for dinner.* This could be a great way to develop more understanding about your diet, and plus, there are few better feelings than making something for your loved ones, especially if it's something you know they'll enjoy.

17. *Visit a park, botanical garden, or wildflower field.* Walking in the park with friends is underrated. Getting out in the fresh air, having a good talk, and looking at the beautiful flowers is a great way to spend a beautiful day.

18. *Play some sports.* Get together to shoot hoops, play soccer, or catch. Even go to the park and toss a Frisbee around.

19. *Check out a comedy club.* Who doesn't love a night of laughing with friends? Keep an eye on the local listings, and the comedians who're coming up. Many comedy clubs post clips on their websites, so you'll get a sense of their humor before you go.

20. *See a movie.* Remember: snacks are totally optional, and unfortunately, most movie snacks aren't very keto friendly. If you must snack while you watch the movie, consider bringing something from home.

21. *Volunteer.* Is there a cause you and a friend feel passionate about? Helping the homeless? Working at an animal shelter? Spending time with the elderly? Either way, volunteering is a great way to spend your time, and you might even meet some new people. You won't have time to think about food. Plus, bonus, you get to feel good about helping people (or animals) all day long, which is a great feeling.

22. *Have a board game night.* This is a great way to spend time with friends. You can have only one game, or several, your choice, and have fun arguing over monopoly.

All in all, you shouldn't let your diet stand in the way of you spending time with the people that you love. Your friends and family should absolutely be your biggest supporters, and when they're not, or they question your decisions, it can be difficult.

The keto diet is still relatively new, and because of this, people often make snap judgments. They hear things like "I don't eat pasta," and they wonder why the heck someone would do that. You might find yourself fending off some comments and advice from people who think they're dietitians or nutritionists and family members who don't understand why you can't eat certain foods you used to love.

The best things to do in these situations are to smile and move on. Remember: many people are insecure about their diet, and they might worry that you'll judge them. Just approach anything that is said negatively about your diet with a "you do you, I do me" approach.

Whatever you do, don't give in. Remember: you're making this journey for a reason, and no matter what that reason is, only you can decide if it's a good enough one. If somebody offers you a piece of cake, and you say no, don't feel bad for saying no, even if it is someone's birthday or a special occasion. It can feel odd being the only one at the table not ordering dessert, but once you see the results, it will all be worth it.

Living With Those Who Aren't into Keto

If you find yourself in a situation where you are living with people who are not into the ketogenic diet, it can be rough. You're trying to partake in this diet, probably experiencing major cravings, and find yourself surrounded by people who are eating all of the foods that you love. You probably won't be able to convince the majority of your housemates to partake in the diet with you, but because we can't all live alone, here are some tips:

- *Tell them your reasons.* Remember: comments from friends and family probably come from a place of genuine concern. When this happens, list out the reasons why you're doing it, show them the science, and ask for their support. They might just be worried that you're not getting the proper amount of nutrition you need.
- *Hide the stuff.* Meaning "don't keep the bad foods in front of you". Keep foods like chips and pasta in a different part of the kitchen, and if you can, avoid cooking with it until you don't crave it anymore. You're more likely to reach for the healthy stuff if it's right in front of you.
- *Replace.* There is an entire list of foods here that you can use to replace some of your favorites, such as zucchini

spaghetti for spaghetti, and introduce recipes that you know that your family will love. Try adding things with a keto twist, and focus on finding foods that not only fit into your guidelines, but you also know they'll like.

Cheating on Keto

Cheating on a diet happens. Everyone gets tempted occasionally, especially when everyone else is around you eating treats that the keto diet restricts. It can also be hard to stop eating foods that you love. It only gets harder when you go out to restaurants or parties, and all you really want is French fries or the delicious crab cakes everyone else is chowing down on.

However, cheating can help you get through it. It can keep you on track. Cheating, or treating yourself, as most people would prefer to call it, can help you do the keto diet without feeling totally deprived. The only issue is that people rarely cheat on diets in the right way. They don't go into cheating with a plan. This guide will not only teach you how to resist cheating but also teach you how to do it the right way. It will help you get back on the horse without too much of an issue and not feel the side effects for too long.

Of course, you shouldn't cheat for the wrong reasons. Things such as peer pressure, politeness, impulsivity, and bad planning are all terrible reasons.

Peer pressure is the worst reason to do anything. We all remember our parents telling us, no matter what, don't give in to peer pressure, right? If people treat you different for your dietary preferences or give their unwanted opinions, just ignore them. Remember why you're doing this; for you, not them. However, it also goes the other way. Don't try to pressure the people around you into trying your diet, and don't be judgmental of people who are choosing to eat differently. Everyone has a different relationship with food, so focus on yours.

Politeness is the second worst reason to do something, especially if it's something you don't want to do. Your Aunt Martha will get over it if you don't eat a piece of her special dessert at the family dinner. If your friend Connor keeps pushing this new recipe on you that he found, but you can't eat it, just remind him of your dietary requirements and tell him that you wish you could. If they keep pushing, just make up the excuse that you have stomach or health issues.

Impulsivity is the worst kind of cheating. If being polite and peer pressure are the worst reasons to cheat, impulsivity is the worst kind of cheating. It just isn't satisfying. It's over too soon, and you don't enjoy it. Planned cheating can make you feel empowered, reminding you that you're in control of what you put in your body and no one else. Impulse cheating leads to you feeling bad about yourself and like you're out of control. It will also lead to no portion control if you just let yourself eat without thinking.

Inadequate planning can also lead to wrong cheating, such as being out and about and realizing that you don't have a way to feed yourself, so you have to settle for a McDonald's burger or a gas station hot dog. Not only have you wasted a cheat card, but it can also feel unsatisfying. To help avoid this, keep a low-carb, high-fat snack in your bag, briefcase, or car, such as nuts. Or keep a list of restaurants you know provide low-carb options in your phone.

There are some more wrong reasons to cheat. Cheating actually can help you stick to your diet. It enables you to avoid feeling so deprived and like you're missing out. You also add some variety and flexibility to your diet. There are also special occasions like holidays or the birthdays of close family members or friends (having birthday cake at the office does not count). If you're heading over to your mom's house for Christmas, and she has the most amazing Christmas cookies ever, it won't hurt to have one. You just need to learn to say no after one. You need to learn how to cheat consciously.

Cheating consciously requires planning, but it also requires knowing what you're getting into. There are some adverse effects. You're opening the door to things like hunger cravings, sugar cravings, weight gain, blood sugar spikes, sickness, and generally feeling terrible. Your mood can suffer, your skin may have a breakout if you are prone to acne, and you can become gassy.

There's also the issue that if you do suffer from sugar addiction, which is very much a real thing, you really can't eat sugar. Sometimes only a little bit will send you over the edge. You really need to ask yourself, "Can I stop at just one?" If you're thinking it's silly to fall into a pattern of sugar addiction, think of it this way: you wouldn't ask an alcoholic only to have one drink, would you?

Now, if you do find yourself tempted to cheat, try some of these tactics to cheat in a way that won't mess up your diet:

- *Delay:* If you're at a party and you really want to try something, eat something else first. Load up your plate with any low-carb options they have, or snack on a prepackaged low-carb snack that you brought along with this very thing in mind. If you still want something after this, tell yourself that you can have it later. Yes, you'll have a piece of chocolate, but you'll have it tomorrow, or when you get home. More often than not, by the time that you're home, you'll probably not even want it anymore.
- *Cheat deliberately:* Plan your cheats, and take charge of them. Write down when you're going to cheat. Set clear boundaries on what you can and cannot eat. For example, maybe you really love hot chocolate, and you really just want one. Instead of going for the large, like you normally do, make a rule for yourself that you only get the small one. You'll feel just as satisfied as if you got the large one, and you can really take your time to savor every sip.
- *Minimize the damage:* Take only small amounts of whatever you're craving. This goes back to ordering the large instead of the small. If you're out with friends, ask if

somebody wants to split a chocolate cake with you instead of someone getting the whole thing, or ask for a bite of theirs. Sometimes just a small bite can really satisfy these cravings.

- *Pick something not high on carbs:* Make a good choice. There are many low-carb keto desserts out there that can be eaten in small portions. Even so, check out the nutritional labels on some of your favorites and find the one with the lower carb count.
- *Cheat after your meal:* Eating fat and protein slows down glucose adsorptions, and will reduce the intensity of your blood sugar spike. It will also help reduce your cravings. You might just be hungry after all.
- *Cheat late:* Cheat after dinner. This limits the window in which your body will go out of low-carb mode, and you will go back into Ketosis overnight. Your body will be burning fat for the rest of the day.
- *Pick something with less sugar:* The ketogenic diet ends up changing your taste buds, as they become more adjusted to eating more whole and healthy foods rather than processed ones. You'll often find that things like candy might taste too sweet. Go for cheats like dark chocolate and low-sugar yogurt.
- *Cheat with fat:* If you're going to cheat on a high-fat diet, make sure you're getting some healthy fats with these cheats. Add butter to bread, fat-rich cream to peaches, and cheese to crackers. You'll find yourself needing fewer carbs to feel satisfied.
- *Cheat with food that matters to you:* Choose foods that you really look forward to having. Like a special family recipe, or if you're in a certain part of town and your favorite bakery is nearby.
- *Cheat before or after workouts:* Cheating right before a workout means that the glucose will be burned off quick, and thus your body will stay in fat burning mode. Cheating after a workout means that you've just burned off whatever

glycogen stores you had. This means that whatever carbs you'll consume will be put back into the glycogen stores, rather than converted to fat. This will help prevent your body from being kicked out of Ketosis.

Getting Back on Track

The most important thing to do after you cheat is to get yourself back on track. This is one of the big reasons why the smart thing to do is to plan your cheats carefully and prepare yourself for the aftermath.

Anticipating Hunger Cravings: be prepared for the fact that after you have a plate of pasta, you might want more. If you anticipate this in advance, you can learn from it and stop yourself from reaching for more.

Learn From Them: keep track of your cheats, and figure out what sets you off and learn from it. You can keep a notebook and write the cheats down, as well as how you feel, what triggers them, and what they bring on in you later.

Forgive Yourself: if you do fall off the wagon, it's OKAY. Yes, it happened, but it's also a learning experience. You can always climb back up from this, and tomorrow is always a new day. It's OKAY. Just keep going. You got this.

Chapter 9: You and Keto

Any big lifestyle change, especially one involving your diet, can be rough. Diet is a big part of our life. We've been eating literally since the day we were born, and we've been doing it every day since.

Why do you want to do the keto diet? That is the first question you need to ask yourself. Do you want to lose weight? Feel less stress? Take control of your health and food intake? Want to have more energy? Whatever it is, this can often drag on. Having a good reason is all well and good at the beginning, but getting yourself in good habits to help you along the way is never a bad thing.

To help yourself get through this diet, here are some useful habits to have to help you tackle these moments where your motivation falters a bit:

Don't call it a diet: This book may be labeled the "keto diet" but don't call it that. It's more like the keto lifestyle, not the diet. While many people consider the keto diet something you can jump on and off without thinking about it too much, this won't work to keep the weight off. If you go straight back to eating the way you were before, you'll just end up right back where you started. Don't consider this something temporary that will last only a year. This is going to be a lifestyle change that will likely follow you for multiple years.

Get a glass of water: We often confuse thirst with hunger. This means that when we're thirsty, we reach for food thinking it will satisfy us. What we really need is water. To drink more water, keep the water in front of you. For example, when you work, put the water bottle on your desk.

Measure your progress: Once a week or month, pull out the measuring tape, grab the scale, and write the new numbers down. Keeping track of your progress will help you stay focused and see how far you've come. Keep in mind that while you'll lose a lot of weight during the first few weeks, afterward, you might find you lose about one pound a week. This is completely normal. If you want to measure by measuring tape, about one inch off your waistline equals to about five pounds of body fat. You could also consider keeping a photo diary, where you photograph yourself topless in the mirror about once or twice a month. Apps like MyFitnessPal will help tremendously.

Get enough sleep: Sleep will help you make better choices. Getting better sleep will stop the stress from affecting your day-to-day judgments and generally make your life better. Lack of sleep also stimulates your appetite, meaning you'll want more food than normal. You won't feel satisfied, and you'll just want to keep eating. Take the time to really get the best sleep, and take a break from the alarm clock once or twice a week.

Pick a Mantra: Did you know that negative thinking changes the chemistry of your brain, and negative thinking attracts more negative thinking? Well, good news: positive thinking does the same thing. People really underestimate the power of positive thinking. Picking a mantra, something like "eat to nourish your body" or "90% kitchen, 10% workout" can help you reach your goals. Repeat it to yourself when you particularly feel down or like you're missing out. Pick one you feel suits your lifestyle the best. Here are some ideas:

- *"Progress not perfection."* If you find yourself feeling like you're not doing everything right, say this to yourself to remember that it's okay not to do everything perfectly the first try. It's also important to remember what works for you rather than what works on everyone else. Focus on what works for you.

- *"Color your plate."* This is a great reminder to fill your plate with lots of colorful vegetables and other healthy foods.
- *"Quality and quantity."* It's not just quality; it's also about how much you eat. Healthy food still has calories, and these calories still add up over time. If you have an issue with overeating, say this to yourself every single time you want to eat more, but you're not hungry.
- *"Every day is new."* If you have a hard time forgiving yourself after a slip-up, this uplifting quote is for you. Reminding yourself that you can always begin again tomorrow is a great way to look at things.

Be Persistent

You need to keep going, even when it feels as if there is no progress being made. Plateaus occur after a while. Real change really only comes with consistency. Real, slow-burning consistency. It can take a while to see real change, but when it does happen, it's pretty incredible.

Stay Motivated

Staying motivated, especially when things like plateaus occur, is very hard. Hitting a plateau sometimes seems akin to hitting a rock wall.

Find a cheering squad: having a social circle who are supportive can be groundbreaking. Not only can they keep you on track, but they can remind you how far you've come, and encourage you. Posting about your journey on social media is a great way to do this. Finding people who are also participating in the keto diet is a great find—mostly thanks to the fact that they'll be able to help you through the rougher parts of the diet. Social media is an incredible thing that enables you to connect with hundreds of millions of people overnight, many of whom are struggling with the same thing. Check out a Facebook group, or the tags on Instagram. Just remember to ignore trolls, vicious internet commenters with nothing nice to say.

Nothing happens overnight: There might be some big changes overnight during the first week, but the likelihood of this keeping up at the same pace is extremely low. Don't be impatient. You might not notice results for nearly six weeks after the initial week.

Keep your goals in minds: Keep them written down somewhere, so you always know where they are and what they are. If you're shopping at the grocery store, keep a little memo in your wallet reminding you why you're heading for the veggies rather than the candy. Keep a list on your fridge of all the reasons you're doing this. Write a list of accomplishments you want to hit, and then as you hit them, tick them off—anything to keep you going.

Make Small Changes

Small habits change everything. Things like drinking more water and learning about nutrition are never something too late to do. And it would be nice if we could just jump into the keto diet without having to worry about completely changing your eating style. However, you might find yourself in way over your head, and all you want to do is eat a giant plate of French fries.

Cutting out foods you love can be tough. There is no shame in taking it easy, at first, and making small changes. This can be anywhere in your journey to a better you—things like taking a nice walk at lunch instead of eating at your desk, and reaching for the veggies and guacamole instead of the regular bag of chips for a snack.

Making small changes benefits you over time because you're turning them into habits. You're replacing the bad habits with the good ones, and instead of depriving yourself, you're whittling them down. Some people out there have gone completely cold turkey, and that works for them, but that might not be for you. You might find yourself relapsing and craving carbs and junk more than ever—not because you want to eat it, but because your body is so dependent on it. Consider just cutting down on your habits, and replacing what's in your fridge with the food you want to eat.

Don't Use Food as Rewards

Rewards specifically imply that you've done something amazing, so why would you choose something that could set you back on your journey? A reward should add to your journey, not make it worse.

What's the point of eating healthy for a week if you just plan on bingeing for a single day by eating whatever you want? Not only will you gain back all the weight you have lost, but you'll also knock yourself right back out of Ketosis, and make the cravings for carbs and sugars worst.

Remember: that sundae you've been thinking about, or the big pizza slice you've been eyeing, will throw you out of Ketosis, rather than being rewarding to you. It will only set you back, moving you right back to first base. Also, thinking of food as rewards can negatively affect your relationship with food by sending you the message that it's only something to be enjoyed on occasion.

Control Emotional Eating

We have all been there. We're bored, tired, stressed, and anxious; you name it, and we end up reaching for the foods that are not good for us. Things like our day-to-day lives can make us feel anxious and alone, and we often reach for food as a way to comfort ourselves. We also reach for food when we have nothing better to do. This needs to stop, not only because it will mess up our macro counting, but it's also not good for us.

Consider these helpful tips:

When stressed: soak in a bath, read a good book, meditate, or do some yoga. Find a healthier way to relax than chowing down.

Low on energy: Your first thought might be to pick up a snack, but if that's not doing it for you, take a walk around the block, listen to some energizing music, or take a short nap. Don't just mindlessly reach for more food—it's likely not the problem.

Lonely or bored: Call a friend and chat for a bit. Take your dog for a walk. Read a book or watch your favorite show on Netflix. Just keep your mind occupied.

Practice Mindful Eating

Mindful eating is when you're just paying attention to your food. You're doing nothing else except eating. This means the following:

- *No distractions.* This means no reading, no watching TV, no driving. This kind of mindless eating will only lead to overeating.
- *Pay attention.* Pay attention to your food. You should; you put a lot of effort into making it. If your mind wanders, keep your attention on your food. Think of it almost like a date that you have to impress.
- *Eat slowly.* It takes time for the signal to reach your brain that you're full. Politeness may have drilled into us that we have to eat everything on our plates, but don't feel too bad. It just means you have leftovers for later!

All in all, that's it! If you follow these healthy tips, you'll be burning those ketones in no time at all!

Conclusion

Congratulations on making it through to the end of *Keto Diet: How to Use the Ketogenic Diet to Lose Weight, Burn Fat, and Increase Mental Clarity, Including How to Get into Ketosis and Fasting on Keto for Beginners*. It should have been informative and provided you with all of the tools you need to achieve your goals, whatever they might be. They can be weight loss, being more focused, building a better life—whatever! You should be able to walk away from reading this knowing where you need to go and that you learned a lot about the keto diet.

The next step is to start the keto diet and keep going. It may be rough for the first few weeks, but it will get better. Track your goals, keep yourself motivated, and really embrace the idea of being a better and healthier you. Your body will be thanking you for years to come, and you'll feel so much better for it.

Remember: you are in control of your diet. You control whether or not you say no to foods that you know are bad for you. You are in control of what foods you stock in your kitchen, what foods you order at a restaurant, how much you eat—everything. You control what goes into your mouth, and you have a right to know what it is doing to your body.

Check out another book by Elizabeth Moore

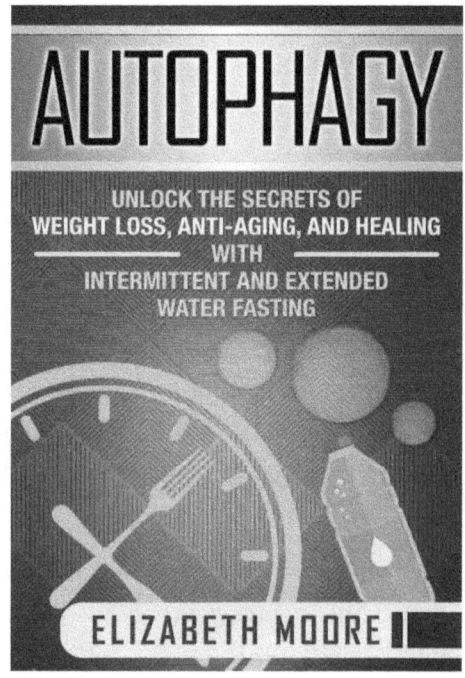

www.ingramcontent.com/pod-product-compliance
Lightning Source LLC
Chambersburg PA
CBHW031149020426
42333CB00013B/587